FACING MYSELF

an introspective look at cosmetic surgery

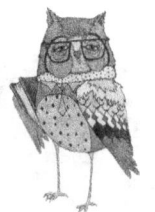

Published by
Our Written Lives of Hope, LLC

Our Written Lives of Hope provides publishing services for authors in various educational, religious, and human service organizations. For information, visit www.OurWrittenLives.com.

All rights reserved. No part of this publication may be reproduced, stored in a retrieval system, or transmitted in any form or by any means, without the permission of the copyright holder.

Copyright ©2016 Rachael Hartman
Cover & Interior Design by Our Written Lives

Library of Congress Cataloging-in-Publication Data
Hartman, Rachael Kathleen 1983
Facing Myself: An Introspective Look at Cosmetic Surgery

Library of Congress Control Number: 2016914389
ISBN: 978-0-9894070-8-3 (paperback)

Scriptures are from various Bible versions, as cited in the text.
Any verse without a citation is the author's rendition.

Chapter 11 is a modified version of work the author wrote for hire. The concepts were first published by LINK247.

FACING MYSELF

an introspective look at cosmetic surgery

Rachael Kathleen Hartman

Dedication

For any person who feels they are "not enough."

Contents

Introduction 7

1: Changing My Face 15

2: Cinderella 25

3: Making the Decision 39

4: I Did It. Now What? 51

5: Hidden Wounds 61

6: The Quest 79

7: Impact on Family 97

8: Privacy, Secrecy, and the Church 117

9: Shamefaced 133

10: Nothing New 143

11: Finding Contentment 161

12: Beautifully Created 179

Afterword 191

About the Author 192

Introduction

A LETTER TO READERS

I just want authentic conversation about cosmetic surgery! Why is it so difficult to find?

I have come to realize that perhaps the topic of cosmetic surgery isn't one most people have thought too deeply about. Maybe it isn't that people are unwilling to talk, but more so that they don't know what to say. It also might be considered a controversial topic.

Many Christians seem incapable of talking about this subject. I have had several people, whom I know love me, warn me not to talk about my surgery to "church people."

One told me, "It's under the blood of Jesus. You don't ever have to bring it up again."

They were supportive, but silenced me with shame. I needed to talk about my experience. As Revelation 12:10-11 says, we overcome the accuser by the blood of the lamb, and the word of our testimony.

For years, I longed for a friend who shared my faith and who would be willing to talk about the cosmetic surgery subject. I consistently met the same spirits: shame and pride.

Some people I've talked to are spiritually ashamed of their surgery; they feel they have to hide it from the Christian world. On the other extreme are people who never had a second thought about their surgery and are confused as to why I think there is something to talk about. It seems they've never had a desire to consider the "why" of their decision, or how it impacts life and relationships.

There is a balanced middle and, thankfully, it's where I find myself today, but I started out in the "ashamed" category. For years after my surgery I kept my "secret" quiet, but I didn't stop thinking about it. I had so much emotional healing work to do, so much to process after my surgery. My desire to talk about it never went away. I had hoped that I could find emotional healing through an authentic community of believers who bear one another's burdens. I couldn't find that community, though I did reach out to many people.

As I attempted to connect with others by sharing my story, I've had a variety of responses to my self-disclosure. I often end up learning about the other person through their response. I've also learned that I still have some insecurities about my body and my surgery choices.

When a person first learns I had plastic surgery, their usual response is, "Really? I can't tell."

I never know exactly what they mean by that. Do they mean, "Really? I can't tell because you still need more." Or is it, "Really? I can't tell; you must have had a great doctor!" Maybe what they mean is, "Really? But you look normal?"

Yes, I look normal, I think to myself. *Did you think cosmetic plastic surgery instantly turns a person into a supermodel?*

Once as I was speaking to a man about how I was writing a book about cosmetic surgery, his eyes immediately drifted to my chest—my small chest. The lines on his face seemed to transform into a question mark.

No, sir. Not there. My face. Hello. Look at my face. Are you listening? I had cosmetic surgery on my face. Breast enhancement isn't the only surgery women choose.

Then there was the woman who responded with, "What did you have done? . . . Oh, it turned out really cute!"

I smiled at her response. I appreciated what she said. She was accepting and unassuming.

After talking to a Christian plastic surgeon I hoped would give me honest feedback about my book, he stared at me with unfeeling eyes and said, "Your nose isn't big anymore. I hope you find healing."

Healing? Really? His response triggered insecurity and defense within me. I felt I had healed. *I know my nose isn't big. I am asking for honest feedback about my writing.*

And then there was the woman speaker I talked to at a conference. Her big focus was overcoming anorexia, so I thought she'd be open to talk about body image. I told her about my book. She said she never thought twice about her surgery and never had one regret, since her breast job made a world of difference in her sexual relationship with her husband.

I listened to her experience, thankful she was willing to share it.

Sometimes people are willing to talk, but they aren't always open to listening. A co-worker once asked, "Why are *you* writing a book on plastic surgery?"

I perceived her tone and the look on her face to be defensive. I was afraid she thought I was coming from a place of judgment. I could only imagine what she might assume. I quickly explained I was writing from personal experience, and a bit of the fear seemed to slide off of her stiff shoulders.

"Oh, that makes sense," she said, abruptly ending the conversation. I had the feeling she would still not be interested in reading my book.

Another co-worker, after slumping her head down for a moment, squared her shoulders and said, "Well, you should talk to *my* plastic surgeon. He goes on mission trips and helps children around the world."

In every one of these interactions, I came to the conversation looking for safe dialogue about an issue that greatly affected my life. Sometimes I found an open heart and listening ears, and other times I regretted sharing my story.

I gained a lot of ground in finding authentic community when I dove into the "recovery world" while writing my first book, *Angel: The True Story of an Undeserved Chance*. I learned about the twelve steps and Biblical principals for emotional healing. Of course, the material was often geared to recovering from substance abuse, but I applied what I learned to find emotional sobriety, and began to build on the concept. Other faith-based programs also helped me admit I had "hurts, habits, and hang-ups" to recover from.

Facing Myself: An Introspective Look at Cosmetic Surgery is not based on recovery steps or principals—as helpful as they were on my journey. Instead, I focus on questions I wish I would have known to ask myself while I was making my (uninformed) decision on whether to go forward with surgery or not.

My experience with cosmetic surgery significantly impacted my life on many levels. I had the power to change my physical body; I did, and my life changed. As my reflection stared back at me in the mirror, I almost didn't recognize her. She was different, but she was still normal. She wasn't perfect. She was still me. I wasn't sure how to feel about her (myself).

It took time for me to grow into my face, but my experience with cosmetic surgery launched me exponentially forward in my personal development. I know I wouldn't be who I am today without the experience. I learned and grew so much. I can't keep what I know to myself.

In 2008, I wrote an anonymous article for a Christian magazine about my experience with elective cosmetic surgery. It was my first attempt at sharing my testimony. Before that time, only my family and a few friends knew about my procedure. The people who knew, even my family, did not understand the full extent of the psychological and emotional issues I experienced—both positive and negative—as a result of my choice. I barely understood what I was going through.

Through the years, I gained perspective on my experience as I sorted through my emotions and learned to treat myself with love and grace. During the process, I felt a range of emotions from happiness, to fear, to shame and doubt, to assurance and acceptance, and finally to contentment.

I wanted to use my journey as a way to help others, so I started writing. This book can be a step in the healing process for people who are hurting like I was. I hope it can help facilitate healing, not from the physical aspect of plastic surgery, but healing for the souls of spiritual and human beings facing similar circumstances. Through writing, I'm able to make sense of my life experiences, including cosmetic surgery. I hope my writing can help someone else make sense of their experiences too.

Choosing to have cosmetic surgery is a very personal choice. If you are considering cosmetic surgery, but have not gone through with it yet, this book can give you insight, and provide you with the tools to make a well-rounded, mature decision about your body. The questions at the end of each chapter will provoke you to dig deep into your heart and discover answers that are true for you.

If you are like me and have already undergone cosmetic surgery, this book will assist you as you process the experience. I hope it will help lead you to find closure on any unresolved issues you may have.

I'm writing this book as a person who chose to have elective cosmetic plastic surgery—not as a person who had reconstructive plastic surgery. There is a difference. Cosmetic surgery is, well, purely cosmetic. Reconstructive plastic surgery rebuilds after a birth defect, cancer, car wreck, or some sort of other physical trauma.

I do not know what it is like to have been born with a physical abnormality, or to have suddenly lost a part of my body due to illness, accident, war, terrorism, or trauma. I can only write about the subject from my own perspective and with the understanding the Lord leads me to.

How does your experience compare to mine? Maybe we are more alike than we know. I want you to know that I respect you and your decisions, and all you've been through. I admire your courage for taking the time to consider your options and weigh them out.

My purpose in writing about cosmetic plastic surgery is not to sway you for or against the idea of undergoing the knife. Rather, it is to examine the issue as a whole from a Christian worldview. I'm writing to challenge you to ask yourself difficult questions, and to give honest answers. I am writing with compassion, healing, grace, and love. I am writing to facilitate bringing God's peace that passes understanding into your thoughts about cosmetic surgery.

Thankfully, over time, the stigma against talking about cosmetic surgery is changing. I have a very dear friend who recently had cosmetic surgery and we've been able to talk about our experiences a bit. **Now, 15+ years after my surgery, I believe it is time for me to begin leading safe and authentic conversations about cosmetic surgery.**

Whether you are aware of it or not, cosmetic surgery and the way we think about it impacts our lives and relationships. Some people like to separate the physical from the spiritual, but I believe all of our experiences are connected. There is an emotional and spiritual component to the physical action taken with cosmetic surgery.

No matter what choice we make—to go forward with cosmetic surgery, or not to—we have many other life choices to make at the same time. We will all have to ask ourselves questions like:

- How will I move forward?
- What will my next choice be?
- What messages will I believe about myself, and what messages will I send to the world?
- What kind of woman (or man) do I want to be?
- How will I actively choose to honor my Creator and serve the world around me?

This book is the beginning of an open dialogue. It's a conversation between friends with hopes, dreams, longings, insecurities, and fears. It's a conversation starter between mothers and daughters, fathers and sons, and between women and men of every race and culture around the world.

♡Rachael Kathleen Hartman

Changing My Face

CHAPTER ONE

I saw myself as having a big nose. I definitely had terribly low self-esteem. I felt inadequate because of my looks and I was tired of feeling that way.

I thought I could solve some of my problems by changing my face. So, as a teenager, I underwent rhinoplasty and chin augmentation—a nose reduction and chin implant—to balance out my facial features.

I thought cosmetic surgery was the answer to stop the hurt inside my heart, but I learned very quickly that was not the case. I soon had to begin the real work of learning to love myself and my imperfections.

I grew up in a preacher's home. My dad was a Chaplain in the U.S. Army and we moved a lot with his career. Through the military, I interacted with a lot of people from various cultures and religions. My family was conservative and I was quite sheltered despite our travels. My parents always empowered my sister, brother, and me to make our own decisions. Mom and Dad always made it clear they loved us and supported us, even if they disagreed with the choices we made.

Despite growing up in a loving Christian home, I still felt I wasn't "good enough." I often compared my looks with the beauty

I saw all around me. I didn't compare myself to the people I saw in magazines or on TV, but with the real-life people I went to school with and interacted with—the people I viewed as beautiful and confident.

I wanted to be beautiful and confident like they were. *If only I had what they had*, I thought. At that time, I couldn't see my own unique talents, passion, and calling. I only saw what I lacked, and I sat on the sidelines watching the people I envied as they lived what I thought was life to the fullest.

My best friend was my minture-runt dachshund, Tuffie. She was my baby from first grade until my second year of college. I still miss her. I took care of her every day. She was five pounds, and epileptic. She was sensitive to my emotions, slept in my bed, and always comforted me.

Growing up, I was very quiet and shy. I also struggled with social anxiety. As a child, my introverted personality gave me the ability to quietly entertain myself and stay focused on school, without drawing much attention. I am still quiet and still have some social anxieties, but my experience today is nothing like it was growing up. Now I have tools to help me cope. Back then, I was overwhelmed.

I didn't have many friends as a kid, and when I did find a friend the friendship would end within a year or so due to our mobile military lifestyle. I learned to be open to meet new people, and to love and appreciate them quickly. I also learned that all relationships, both good and bad, would come to an end at some point—probably sooner than later. I would be leaving within six months to three years, and most of the time it wasn't worth the effort to try to make friends. It was just too difficult to care about other people when I knew I would be moving soon, and would never see them again.

When Dad got orders, we all got orders. From my childhood perspective, I was a good soldier. I had very strong feelings of patriotism, a love for my God and country. I viewed my life as an act of service. I still feel that way. My lifestyle taught me that duty came first, and that I had to soldier-on through inner pain.

I spent most of my childhood and teenage years looking forward to the day when I would find the place where I belonged. It was a place I dreamed of where I was accepted, had many friends, and could live happily for the rest of my life. I was sure that I would find my place, fall in love, and have a family of my own. I dreamed of the day I'd meet that special person who would accept and love me for who I was.

As years passed, I became tired of waiting to find where I belonged. *There must be something wrong with me*, I thought. *I must not be good enough. Why do the girls my age treat me so badly? Why isn't Prince Charming searching for me? Why am I always alone? Why doesn't anyone notice me?* I concluded there must be something wrong with me. It was the only thing that made sense. There was no alternative in my mind.

Despite my loneliness and low self-esteem, I never stopped living for God. I loved the Lord with all of my heart. He's been the Love of my life who has never left me. He's accepted me with all of my inadequacies and imperfections. I am very sure if it hadn't been for the love and grace of God being so real and powerful in my life, I would have been very lost in this world. I cannot say where I would be, probably on the streets somewhere, if not for the love of God.

But God's love wasn't enough for me. I wanted love and attention from a person. I was willing to do whatever it took to get that love, as long as I could get by with it Biblically as a Christian. I recognized my vulnerability and decided it was safer to close myself off emotionally. Due to fear of becoming a statistic and running to men for love, I withdrew socially and poured myself into pursuing God and ministry.

Still, thoughts of inadequacy plagued me. Maybe if I were a nicer person, maybe if I followed all of the rules, excelled in education, and prayed more—maybe then I'd find acceptance and love. In all of my longing, I missed God's true desire, which was for me to accept others and to love the unloved, instead of waiting for everyone else to accept and love me.

My plan backfired. I became such a "super-Christian" I was untouchable. I was so busy trying to be a better person I failed to live life. I didn't have the skills to build lasting relationships. I found myself lonely and falling into old patterns of thought. *It is me. There is something wrong with me.* I defined myself by my imperfections.

In my mind, I had to change something about myself, so I would be worthy of love. I believed that lie, and manifested the belief through various parts of my life. I changed the way I dressed to please the people at whatever church I happened to be attending.

I fixed my hair the way they fixed their hair. I chose glasses I saw other people wearing. I repressed my personality, ignored my heart-cries, and focused on pleasing others.

It wasn't a new concept for me to want to change myself in hope of gaining love and acceptance. When I was ten and someone commented that I was chunky, I determined I would lose weight. My uneducated ten-year-old mind had no idea how to diet. Without anyone knowing, I began to limit my food and started constantly thinking about how I looked. By the time I was fourteen I began exercising a lot. In my mind, unless I made it to a size 4, I would not be thin enough. I never made it down that small—I liked to eat too much, but I was still consumed by my looks and obsessed with ensuring I stayed thin.

I was never diagnosed with an eating disorder, though my parents voiced their concerns of it when I was in high school. I did not go to extremes to lose weight. I hated throwing up, so I never attempted to binge and purge that way, but I still had a problem. I believed my entire worth depended on how I looked. I even believed that God would love me less if I wasn't perfectly modest and holy, which my church emphasized.

I may have never been diagnosed with an eating disorder, but I knew I struggled with negative self-image, striving for perfection, and limiting my food. When I was ready to hear and accept it, I learned that over-exercise was a form of bulimia. I was purging through exercise along with not eating healthy foods.

I remember the day I decided I was tired of being hungry. I was in Bible college, and it was several years after my cosmetic facial surgery. I placed one hand on the front of my stomach and one hand on my back. I felt nothing but hollow inside. From that point on, I began to focus on healthy eating and moderate exercise.

I turned seventeen the summer I decided to pursue cosmetic plastic surgery. I knew I had a problem in the way I felt about myself. I felt horrible inside and I wanted to change. I prayed about going forward with plastic surgery. I even fasted about it. I cried and sorted through my thoughts. Before I had the surgery, I came to a place where I was at peace with God and myself concerning my choice. I believed I had the "OK" from God to have surgery.

A few days before I went to the hospital, I told my sister I was becoming a stronger person by having plastic surgery because I finally accepted the fact that I was not perfect, and was going to do something about it. At that time, I couldn't see that I was still on a quest for unattainable perfection. It was true, however, that I was stepping out and trying something new. Taking that risk was one of the best—and most challenging—choices I've made.

I don't regret my surgery. It helped make me the person I am today. I grew as a person because I took a risk and made a change. My choice wasn't easy. I suffered a great deal of physical pain, including nerve damage I still feel at times.

After the surgery, for a few years, I continued to struggle emotionally with the same low-self esteem issues I had before my surgery. Cosmetic surgery didn't make me perfect, and it didn't fix my emotional problems. Instead, it forced me to see myself for who I was. It helped me to accept myself, despite my imperfections.

I've never met anyone who has ever guessed that I had cosmetic surgery on my face. Most people are surprised when I tell them, because I look very natural. I'm not a supermodel or mainstream beautiful. I'm an average pretty person. My nose is still not perfect. In fact, it is a little uneven, and pictures of my side profile are still not the most flattering.

I am thankful I had a good surgeon. I've heard many stories of surgeries gone wrong that left the patient longing for their pre-surgery self. I've had those feelings too, but not because of a botched job. I found myself wondering what I would have looked like as an adult, fully grown into my face, if I had not had surgery.

What would my personal development journey have looked like if I had pursued a healthy self-image without changing my face surgically? I've wondered what I would have been like had I experienced secure and close friendships before my surgery. Would I have made the same choices if I had the emotional and relational stability I longed for?

My journey has not been easy. I've faced many questions and challenges after my surgery. I've suffered in silence in cold weather, not being able to feel parts of my face, and not feeling comfortable to talk about it to anyone. I've worried that some day I'd meet a guy and fall in love, only to be rejected once he found out I had changed the face God gave me. I began driving myself crazy worrying about possible rejection.

Several years after my surgery, I decided to start talking about it. I thought it would be easier to be open about who I am and what I had done—to just be real from the start—instead of hiding it, and fearing rejection. I still didn't tell many people about my surgery; it's not something that comes up in daily conversation. But talking about it helped in my healing process.

I don't think about my surgery every day like I did when it first happened. My identity is no longer wrapped up in the fact that I had surgery. I still have body features I like and some I don't like, but I don't obsess anymore. I stopped obsessing years ago.

It's been over fifteen years since my surgery. I'm not the same person I was back then, but my experiences helped shape who I am today. I realize the decisions I make today will stay with me for the rest of my life, just like yesterday's decisions are with me now.

There is no going back when it comes to body alteration, just like there is no going back when it comes to drugs, relationship choices, overeating, getting into debt, or anything else. We must take responsibility for our decisions, and move forward. We can't change the past. We must climb out of the place we've dug ourselves into, and when we are free, we will find gratefulness because we have lived, survived, and overcome.

Whatever journey you are on, whatever the reason you are reading this book, my prayer for you is to find God's grace. I pray God grants you the grace to love yourself, your family members, your friends, your church, your community, and everyone you meet. I pray God's grace would infuse your heart with love and compassion so you will take the time to listen to other people and take them seriously.

Your life matters. My life matters. Everyone's life matters. The choices we make matter. The future of our children and our country matters. The way we view life and each other matters.

It matters because there is more to our lives than what we can see. There is an eternity waiting for each of us. There is a God who gave Himself for us, to save us from ourselves and the hurt and pain of this world.

He is our Creator and what He thinks matters. What He made matters. And the way we approach this life and these bodies He has given us matters as well.

1 Corinthians 6:19-20 NLT

Don't you realize that your body is the temple of the Holy Spirit, who lives in you and was given to you by God? You do not belong to yourself, for God bought you with a high price. So you must honor God with your body.

Questions for Reflection

- How is your relationship with the Creator God?
- How is your relationship with yourself?
- Do you love yourself and your body?
- Does the way you feel about yourself keep you from engaging in relationships that are good for you?
- Do you treat your body with respect as the temple of the Holy Ghost?
- Do you change yourself in order to please other people?
- Do you feel worthy of love and acceptance, even with your imperfections?

Cinderella

CHAPTER TWO

Cinderella. Everyone knows Prince Charming is seeking his true love. She is the woman who perfectly fits the glass slipper. Unlike the Disney cartoon version of the story most of us are familiar with, in the original Grimm Brothers' tale, the first evil stepsister cut off her toe to make her foot fit the shoe. The second stepsister cut off her heel to make her foot fit.

"The impulse to alter appearance may be differentially defined and executed by women around the globe, but there is a commonly held wish or belief that changing the body will magically change relationships."[1] I read that quote by H.S. Edelman in an article in the *Journal of Popular Culture*. There is much research available on cosmetic surgery and the reasons people pursue body alteration.

A *USA Today* article, titled *Why People Want Plastic Surgery*, reported approximately 70 percent of people seeking elective cosmetic plastic surgery said they hoped for emotional and psychological benefits, including happiness, self-esteem, and confidence. Another 45 percent, mostly men, hoped for the benefit of being socially accepted and attractive.[2]

Many people do experience a boost in self-esteem after cosmetic surgery, as long as they consider their surgery a success. Particularly, people who are born with physical abnormalities, or have deformities due to trauma, may feel their lives have been positively transformed after plastic surgery. Plastic surgery can be a therapeutic stop on the road to emotional recovery after living a life feeling different from everyone else.

But are we *really* that different from everyone else, even with our imperfections and without surgery?

Cultural beauty standards influence social acceptance and our perception of normality. It's not a new idea. Art has always communicated ideal beauty. From the days of cave drawings depicting hunters and warriors, to Michelangelo's sculptures and paintings of the ideal human form, art and its immortalized beauty influences us.

The invention of the camera in 1839 led to the eventual mass circulation of fashion magazines, which started in the late 1800s. Cameras made it possible to communicate ideal beauty to larger audiences more than ever before. In the 20s, 30s, and 40s, Hollywood movies impacted the cultural definition of the standard American beauty. Thus the conflict, and another quote from Edelman, **"With standards comes confusion: [we] want to be individually distinctive, but [to also] comply with norms."**[3]

Sociologists recognize the aftermath of mass media and cultural beauty norms as seen in society's level of body image satisfaction. Girls, ages 5 to 7, exhibited lower self-esteem and a greater desire for thin bodies after exposure to ultra-thin Barbie dolls.[4] Research documents two mental processes involved when women are exposed to media models. The first mental process is imagination—dreaming of being the model. The second mental process is comparison—how does my form compare to the model's?

I don't have to convince anyone that American popular culture pressures people to be "beautiful" in order to be accepted or worthy of love. There are many movements today that seek to change cultural beauty ideals as promoted by the fashion industry. Many people from a diverse backgrounds and educational levels agree that an emotionally negative response results from the American standard of beauty. Organizations, such as The Dove Movement for Self-Esteem, work to bring attention to this important issue. These groups are motivated to prevent eating disorders and body image issues resulting from comparing normal healthy bodies to digitally enhanced photographs.

The good news is that these groups are doing a great job of getting the message out. More than ever before, we are aware of digital photography enhancements. There is an openness and idea sharing coming from creative professionals as they seek to connect to their audience, sharing techniques and the behind-the-scene process. The average person now has access to computer software such as Photoshop, free online photo editor websites, and apps for smartphones that allow us to digitally manipulate pictures.

With more and more access to the "how" behind the beautiful images we see, we can understand "why" our untouched photos don't make us look like models—because even models don't look like models in untouched photos. Reality TV shines light on the humanity behind the celebrities. YouTube video tutorials show us how to manipulate images, and apply make-up to completely change our look. We understand with our minds that no one looks perfect—unless artistically altered. But is that knowledge transferring into our hearts?

Even with all of our knowledge, millions of people are not only altering their photographs, they are altering their bodies. If we want to change our bodies, we have access to surgeons that will change us. It's like Photoshop in real-life. The truth of the matter is that plastic surgery was not as common in its origins as it is today. It's now becoming a fad, like going on a diet or dying hair, but it didn't start out that way.

The History of Plastic Surgery[5]

Plastic surgery has been around for about 120 years. In its beginning, the plastic surgery movement was noble and altruistic across the board. The first recorded breast augmentation surgery was in 1895 when surgeons transplanted back tissue into a woman's breast in order to correct asymmetry. In 1899, doctors injected beeswax, paraffin and vegetable oil into breasts as the first implants.

The field of plastic surgery grew from 1910 to 1919 during World War I, as doctors treated wounded soldiers and performed the first skin grafts. In 1924, Johns Hopkins University opened the first U.S. plastic surgery training program. From 1930 to 1939, plastic surgeons and emergency room doctors worked together to bring attention to the high rate of facial injuries during car accidents. Their advocacy resulted in car manufacturers developing shatterproof windshields, and many other safety features now required in cars.

In the 1940s, during World War II, the military opened nine plastic surgery centers to focus on treating burns and facial trauma caused by trench warfare. In the 50s, Surgeon Ralph Millard introduced techniques for correcting cleft palate and cleft lips. His research was later nominated for a Pulitzer Prize. Thousands of patients received treatment for facial deformities in the 50s. Plastic surgeon Joseph Murray performed the first live organ transplant in 1954 for a kidney patient. He earned a Nobel Prize for his work in 1990.

In the 1960s, surgeons began using silicone for breast implants. Over the next twenty years, advancement in plastic surgeries for both facial surgery and breast augmentation produced successful results for both reconstructive and cosmetic patients. In 1982, surgeons began offering liposuction to U.S. patients after techniques were initially developed in France. From 1990 to 1999, over 1.2 million reconstructive surgeries and 1 million cosmetic surgeries occurred in the U.S., including the first successful hand transplant in 1999.

In 1992, the Food and Drug Administration ruled silicone breast implants unsafe, which left saline implants as the only option for breast enhancement. In 1998, President Bill Clinton approved a law requiring insurance companies to pay for reconstructive breast augmentation after mastectomies due to cancer. From 2000-2009, plastic surgeons advocated for laws that required insurance to pay for treatment and reconstruction of birth deformities. Around that time, doctors introduced body contouring to remove extra skin after major weight loss.

In 2005, French plastic surgeons performed the first partial face transplant. In 2008, German medical professionals successfully completed the first double arm transplant on a 54-year-old man who received arms from a 19-year-old donor. In Spain in 2010, a team of 30 surgeons performed the first full-face transplant.

Statistics[6]

Though some plastic surgeons focus specifically on trauma patients or reconstructive needs, many plastic surgeries in the U.S. occur for purely cosmetic reasons. Between 1964 and the early 1990s, approximately 2 million women hired medical professionals to permanently augment the size of their breasts via silicone implants. Of those women, only 20 percent had the surgery for reconstruction post-mastectomy. The remaining 80 percent chose breast augmentation as a purely cosmetic surgery.[7]

The number of people choosing elective procedures grows every year. Even in the midst of economic crisis, there were 1.7 million surgical cosmetic procedures in 2015, including breast augmentation, liposuction, nose reshaping, eyelid surgery, tummy tucks, and more. In addition, there were 5.8 million reconstructive procedures, including tumor removals, maxillofacial surgery, scar revision, hand surgery, and laceration repair.

Of the total number of overall U.S. cosmetic surgical procedures in 2015, 87 percent, or 1.5 million cosmetic surgeries, were performed on women. Only 207,869 surgeries were for men.

For men, nose reshaping was the most common cosmetic surgery with 53,248 reported cases. Compare that number to the number of total hair transplants for men, which was only 11,366. Men only make up 13 percent of cosmetic surgery patients.

Ethnically, Caucasians make up the majority of all cosmetic surgery recipients, with 10.9 million patients in 2015. Hispanics make up the next highest ethnic group at 1.7 million cosmetic procedures, followed by African Americans at 1.4 million, and Asian Americans at 1.1 million. The American Society of Plastic Surgeons reports the following distribution of surgeries by age, and most common procedure for each age group.

2015 Cosmetic Surgical Procedures by Age[8]

Age	# of	1st Most Common	2nd Most Common
13-19	64,470	Nose Reshaping	Breast Augmentation
20-29	249,243	Breast Augmentation	Nose reshaping
30-39	365,138	Breast Augmentation	Liposuction
40-54	543,274	Eyelid surgery	Liposuction
55+	373,418	Eyelid surgery	Face-lift

2015 Popular Surgeries[9]

There were 1,706,106 total cosmetic surgical procedures in the U.S. in 2015. These numbers do not include minimally invasive procedures such as Botox, only surgical procedures.

My surgery happened in the year 2000, just before I entered my senior year of high school. I found statistics showing the change in percentage in the number of surgeries from 2000 to 2015. Breast augmentation is up by 31 percent. The two procedures I had done were chin augmentation (down by 35 percent), and nose reshaping, which is also called rhinoplasty (down by 44 percent).

The most recent statistics available show that breast augmentation is still the number one surgery in the U.S. with 279,143 enhancements (implants) in 2015. Of the enhancements, 7,840 were for girls between the ages of 13-19. There were 79,640 implants for young women between the age of 20-29. The highest number, 102,585 were for women ages 30-39 years old. The numbers decline as we go up in age. 82,251 were for women aged 40-54, and 6,827 were for women aged 55 and older.

The statistics listed implant removals separately (24,661), as well as breast lifts (99,614), aesthetic breast reduction in women (40,650), and breast reduction in men (27,456). That's a total of 471,524 people living in the United States that had a cosmetic procedure on their breasts last year. It's very likely you know at least one of those people, and you may be one of them yourself.

The next highest numbers for cosmetic surgical procedures in 2015 were as follows: liposuction (222,051), nose reshaping

(217,979), eyelid surgery (203,934), and a tummy tuck (127,967). Recently, the trend is turning to cosmetic surgery on genitalia (no statistics are available from the ASPS) and buttocks (between 2,500 and 14,000 depending on the procedure).

The Pressure is On

No doubt, life is full of pressure to look a certain way regardless of what culture, ethnicity, or religion a person is. Young girls in particular often feel the need to conform to model standards. I believe the motives behind current plastic surgeries vary between genuine physical need and displaced emotional and social need.

Christian girls and women are not immune to the pressure to conform. In fact, they have pressure from two sides concerning the way they look. There is the pressure to be beautiful by society's standards, and the pressure to be "modest" and "holy" by the church's standards. The spiritual battle is intense, and there are many untended wounds in hearts all around us.

Few escape the pandemic pressure to conform in some way or another in order to be accepted. Some may change the way they dress or style their hair. Others may take more drastic measures and surgically change a body feature. The point is, we feel like we have to change the outside to be accepted and that is a problem.

Sadly, many men and women around the world fight for their life as they battle low self-esteem, eating disorders, and now, addiction to plastic surgery. The problem is far reaching and debilitating.

They are trapped and unable to see how much they could help their fellow man, if only they knew their worth.

Is plastic surgery the answer? Cut away the fat, cut away the extra, and maybe someone out there will see me for who I am? Cut away the ugly, cut away the shameful, and maybe someone out there will love me? If I looked better, I'd have the confidence to speak out on issues. If I was a better person, maybe God could use me in some kind of ministry. If I felt better about myself, I could love others. These lies too often limit us from reaching out and making our world a better place.

I read about an 18-year-old girl that died after a bad reaction to anesthesia during her breast augmentation surgery. I can't help but think of the **30,246 girls under the age of 18 who had nose reduction surgery in 2015**, and the 7,840 girls under the age of 18 who had breast enhancements that same year.

Like me, these girls had emotional and spiritual reasons for making the decision they made. How many of those girls died? I don't know. Was the risk of plastic surgery worth it? To those girls, yes, the benefit was worth risking their life.

If you are considering plastic surgery, I am not trying to stop you, but I want you to be aware of the risks involved. Plastic surgery may be the right thing for you. It is your decision, and I hope that you make it for yourself, and do not make your decision based on what culture tells you about beauty. Plastic surgery may make your quality of life better. It may ease a physical strain or correct a defect that impacts your daily life. I didn't choose plastic surgery because of a physical problem. I chose it because I thought I was ugly. I challenge you to be honest about why you want cosmetic surgery.

I believe we can make the greatest difference for Christ in our world if we believe He can use us. At the time I chose to have a cosmetic procedure done, I had very low self-esteem. I could not see how God could use me. I could not see my worth. My low self-esteem had a direct impact on my choice for surgery. I didn't make my choice based on hoping for a positive outcome. I made it trying to escape a negative emotional state of mind.

If you have low self-esteem, I encourage you to do what it takes to overcome the negative and gain a positive self-image before you consider plastic surgery. Changing the outside won't change the inside.

Did I overcome my low self-esteem? Yes, but plastic surgery didn't do it for me. I had to work for it with the help of the Holy Spirit, and I still have to work to maintain healthy self-esteem. It's a lot easier now. When those old thoughts and feelings come up, I put a stop to them immediately—I will never go back to living life feeling worthless. God has shown me my worth and no one can take that away.

Song of Solomon 4:7 ESV

You are altogether beautiful, my love; there is no flaw in you.

Questions for Reflection

- What surgery are you considering, or what surgery did you already undergo?
- Why are you considering, or why did you choose, plastic surgery?
- How do you, or did you, believe surgery would change your life?
- Do you have healthy self-esteem?
- Did anyone else encourage you toward cosmetic surgery, or was it your idea?
- How will plastic surgery change your quality of life?
- Do you have the support of your family, friends, church, counselor, doctor, or others concerning your decision?

Endnotes

1   Edelman, H. S. (1994). Why is Dolly Crying? An Analysis of Silicone Breast Implants in America as an Example of Medicalization. *Journal Of Popular Culture, 28*(3), 19-32.

2   Why People Want Plastic Surgery. (2005). *USA Today Magazine, 134*(2725), 2.

3   Edelman, H. S. (1994). Why is Dolly Crying? An Analysis of Silicone Breast Implants in America as an Example of Medicalization. *Journal Of Popular Culture, 28*(3), 19-32.

4   Helga Dittmar (2009). How Do "Body Perfect" Ideals in the Media Have a Negative Impact on Body Image and Behaviors? Factors and Processes Related to Self and Identity. Journal of Social and Clinical Psychology: Vol. 28, Special Issue: Body Image and Eating Disorders, pp. 1-8.

5 PlasticSurgery.org
6 Ibid.

7   Edelman, H. S. (1994). Why is Dolly Crying? An Analysis of Silicone Breast Implants in America as an Example of Medicalization. *Journal Of Popular Culture, 28*(3), 19-32.

8 PlasticSurgery.org
9 Ibid.

Making the Decision

CHAPTER THREE

Before I made the decision to go forward with cosmetic surgery, I took several months to consider whether or not I really wanted surgery. I prayed about it. I searched my heart and I asked God to guide me in my decision. Ultimately, I based my choice on the fact that it was what I wanted. I was not able to objectively consider *why* I wanted to change my face. I just followed my heart.

Though I felt I had the "OK" from God to go forward, I didn't receive a direct word or confirmation that He gave me His stamp of approval for plastic surgery. I also didn't receive a stop sign. God was with me throughout the decision-making process, but He let me make my own decision. Through it all, He never left me and He is still here loving me.

Jeremiah 17:9 KJV
*The heart is deceitful above all things,
and desperately wicked: who can know it?*

One article I read compared elective plastic surgery to making an expensive purchase. The writer shared an observation from a successful salesman. He said 10 percent of a sale is based on the buyer's analytical judgment, and 90 percent is based on emotion.[1] I personally try not to make financial purchases based on emotion. I don't go shopping just to see what I can find that I might like to buy. I go shopping with a purpose for a specific item.

If I end up seeing something I like, I leave the store without it. If I am still thinking of the item a few days later, I know I really want it, and the purchase won't be based on momentary emotion. Taking a step back to allow emotions time to settle is a good idea when it comes to making a decision about cosmetic surgery.

Once I decided to have surgery, I met with the surgeon one time. He touched my face, my nose and my chin, as if he were feeling for any lumps or abnormalities in the skin. We talked briefly, but I was never asked to take any psychological assessment or to attend any counseling appointments. (Years later, of my own choice, I did seek out and attend counseling sessions in which I discussed emotional and relational issues which influenced my choice to have surgery.)

I remember feeling shy as I met with the surgeon. I must have been very anxious because I do not remember anything he asked me that day. I do remember he said he would focus on the bottom part of my nose and would place an implant in my chin to balance out my facial structure.

The surgery I had on my nose is called rhinoplasty. It's a procedure that reshaped the bottom cartilage area of my nose. The upper portion of my nose was not changed. My nose was not broken during my procedure and my nasal cavity was not packed with wound dressing, which happens in the more extensive septorhinoplasty where the nasal septum (cartilage between the nostrils) is altered.

The day of the surgery, I spoke with an anesthesiologist who asked me a few typical questions. It was a day procedure, which did not take long to perform. I only stayed at the hospital a few hours in the recovery room waking from sedation. I do not recall having any follow up appointments.

Deciding to undergo cosmetic surgery was the first major decision I made for myself. It was the first choice that I had to live with, and commit to, no matter what. There was no going back regardless of the outcome.

At the time, I did not understand the risk I was taking with my life and my face. I do not believe I was experienced enough as a sixteen-year-old to make an informed decision about plastic surgery, but I do not regret my decision because I learned so much through the experience.

Though I am happy with the results, the surgery itself and the changes to my face are minimal compared to the inward emotional and personal growth I experienced as I continued to mature. When I made the choice to undergo cosmetic surgery, I took a risk. In doing so, I gained a life experience that is worth more to me than the surgery itself. I learned so much from it, and I'm still learning.

I did not become addicted to cosmetic surgery and I have no desire to have cosmetic surgery again. I did, however, continue my addiction to pursing unrealistic and ideal perfection in many other areas of my life. I still have to consciously commit to trusting God when I feel I've failed, and when I feel unworthy of love due to imperfections.

I wonder how long it would have taken me to grow emotionally to the point I am today if I had not had surgery. Did my decision help me to mature and work through my insecurities faster than I would have without surgery? I believe it did. I experienced rapid growth and transitioned to a place of healthier self-esteem, not because I looked different, but because of the lessons I learned. I learned that changing my looks didn't change me. I learned to accept myself and come to a place of thankfulness for my imperfections.

Should You Choose Cosmetic Surgery?

Deciding if you should pursue cosmetic surgery is a very personal choice. You are the only one that has to live in your body. You have one life, and you make the decisions on how you live it. You have the freedom to choose, but you don't have the power to select the consequences of your choice. When you're knocked out under anesthesia on the operating table, you are completely out of control of what happens. You must trust your surgeon (who is, albeit, a trained professional) with your life, your looks, and your potential self-image.

How much self-esteem are you expecting your surgeon to give you? How much responsibility are you taking in obtaining a healthy self-image? What is it you hope to receive as the payout for surgery—an emotional high, self-admiration, or an ideal body feature? Are you asking too much of your surgeon?

In this chapter, I'm going to discuss how plastic surgery could potentially interact with your mental health and your overall wellbeing. It is important that you take into consideration deep-rooted psychological and relational needs that may be driving your choices. Any reason—outside of a physical, medical, or bodily condition—which is influencing your choice toward cosmetic surgery, will remain an issue after the surgery is over.

Cosmetic Surgery and Psychological Health

Though surgeons are encouraged to evaluate patients for potentially conflicting psychiatric issues before agreeing to perform cosmetic surgery, as a whole the medical field is not based on psychological research. **Plastic surgeons are generally not trained in psychology; they are trained to treat physical problems with physical answers.** Over time, various psychologists' ideas have influenced the educational system that trains plastic surgeons, and have brought more attention to the psychological health of surgery candidates.

Throughout the decades, psychologists have offered varied opinions about the impact of plastic surgery on the mind. In 1925, Dr. Sigmund Freud recommended psychotherapy for women seeking cosmetic surgery because he deemed them suffering from the "common female feeling" of worthlessness.

In 1960, psychoanalyst John Gedo refined Freud's view and said cosmetic surgery was the same as taking a pill or going to psychotherapy to improve self-esteem.[2] In 1975, research showed most cosmetic surgery patients were people who suffered with inferiority or frustration due to a physical abnormality, not someone whose main goal was seeking beauty.[3]

Currently, psychologists are concerned with plastic surgery as an addictive disorder, as well as viewing it as a result of other diagnostic disorders. Despite concerns from mental health professionals, most surgeons are not trained to assess or diagnose psychological issues and may not be fully aware of what is motivating their patients toward surgery.

In 2002, psychologists developed a simple questionnaire for surgeons to use to assess patients for psychological morbidity before an operation.[4] Most surgeons now require patients to complete a mental health questionnaire, or see a counselor or psychologist before a cosmetic surgery is approved.

Cosmetic surgeons are advised not to operate on patients who are depressed, obsessive compulsive, uncooperative, or who have unrealistic expectations.[5] In accordance with the Hippocratic Oath to "do no harm," doctors cite social perfectionism and major life events, such as divorce, as reasons to refuse to treat patients with plastic surgery procedures. Dr. Ronald G. Wheeland, M.D., who at one time was the president of the American Academy of Dermatology, said he considers it a red-flag if a patient wants cosmetic surgery in order to please another person.

Many people believe plastic surgery benefits mental health, but there is no research that supports that theory. Plastic surgery recipients are actually found more likely to have neurosis and personality disorders, as well as substance abuse problems.[6]

Results from five research studies with over 37,000 U.S. and Canadian participants, found cosmetic surgery patients two to three times more likely to commit suicide than the average person.[7] In particular, women with breast implants were 73 percent more likely to commit suicide than the general population.[8]

Body Dysmorphic Disorder (BDD), also called imagined ugliness, is a common trait among people who choose cosmetic surgery. People with BDD obsess over what they consider to be physical flaws, usually features others would deem nonexistent or barely noticeable. One study found approximately 2.5 percent of American college-aged women suffered from BDD. A German study showed between 1 and 2 percent of the country's general population met criteria for a BDD diagnosis. A person with BDD is 45 times more likely to commit suicide than the average person, a suicide rate more than double that of people with major depression, and three times higher than the suicide rate for people with Bipolar Disorder.[9]

Plastic Surgery as an Addiction

I believe we are all vulnerable to addictions of some sort. We can be addicted to relationships, people pleasing, lust, power, money, gambling, drugs, food, exercise, work, TV, adrenaline pumping activities, and even religious performance. We can turn to any number of activities and experiences to try to fill the void inside our hearts created by legitimate unmet needs for love and acceptance.

Just like everything else in life, plastic surgery can lend itself to addictive behavior. Perhaps it's an addiction to an ideal body image a person is willing to do anything to obtain. Not everyone who chooses plastic surgery becomes addicted—just like not everyone who drinks alcohol becomes an alcoholic, but it is a prominent concern to be aware of.

Researcher Amnon Suissa wrote about a woman who underwent seven cosmetic surgeries by the time she was 27. To pay for the procedures, the woman went into major debt—maxing out her credit cards, stealing money from her friends and family, and eventually selling her body by posing for pornographic pictures. The woman was hurting emotionally, and suffering from relational issues. She pursued aesthetic bodily perfection to distract from family problems, and alleviate low self-esteem.[10]

Plastic surgery becomes an addiction when a person is never satisfied with their body, and continues down a road of destructive behaviors in order to pursue ideal body image through surgery. Taking out loans they cannot repay, selling themselves through prostitution or porn, burglary, and engaging in illegal and dangerous activities to make money are just some of the destructive behaviors addicts use to obtain the money to pay for plastic surgery.[11]

Addiction to plastic surgery can be just as dangerous and destructive as an addiction to drugs. In many ways plastic surgery addiction can be even more destructive than drugs because there aren't a lot of people aware of the harmful issues surrounding it. H.S. Edelman put it this way, "With our mania for surgery in this country, we seem to have blurred the distinction between toning up at the gym and having our thighs liposuctioned; between having a facial and a face lift... It is not the same thing, folks. Surgery can kill you. And for many women it becomes addictive."[12]

Normalization and Promotion of Cosmetic Surgery

The choice to pursue cosmetic surgery is often a reflection of a person's relationship with themselves and their social support system. It is also indicative of a culture that over-medicalizes all areas of life. There is a problem when we focus on altering the physical body with drugs and other medical procedures as an answer for problems that are social, emotional, and spiritual in nature.[13]

America is not the only country where cosmetic surgery is popular—it's a worldwide fad. It surprised me to learn how widespread and accepted cosmetic surgery is in countries such as Venezuela, Argentina, South Korea, and even Iran. Each individual has personal reasons for considering plastic surgery, and each culture has social reasons for normalizing the behavior.

Venezuela and Argentina both place high value on physical appearance. In those countries, plastic surgery is free and available to young people who receive authorization from a doctor or psychologist. In Iran, some women pursue plastic surgery as an act of exerting power over their own bodies—perhaps an act of defiance against oppressive androcentrism? Many females in South Korea see plastic surgery as an economic investment, hoping to enhance beauty and make themselves more competitive in gaining a wealthy husband.[14]

Questions for Reflection

- Who are you considering as your plastic surgeon? Have you researched your surgeon? Do you trust them with your life?
- Does your doctor show care or concern for your mental, emotional, and physical wellbeing?
- Have you completed a psychological assessment or seen a counselor regarding cosmetic surgery?
- Are you willing to talk to a professional psychologist or counselor about your motivations and decision-making process regarding cosmetic surgery?
- Do you struggle with addiction in other areas of your life?
- Have you ever experienced symptoms of BDD, or had thoughts of suicide?
- Are there any underlying issues you need to resolve before making a decision about cosmetic surgery?
- Have you made any decisions in your past that you had to live with regardless of the outcome?
- What are the possible consequences (positive and negative) that could impact your life and wellbeing if you go through with plastic surgery? Is it worth the risk for you to proceed?
- Study Psalm 139. What is God speaking to your heart about His love for you?

Endnotes

1 Clodius, L. L. (2002). "The importance of recognizing body dysmorphic disorder in cosmetic surgery patients: do our patients need a preoperative psychiatric evaluation?" by V. Vindigni et al. *European Journal Of Plastic Surgery*, 25(6), 309. doi:10.1007/s00238-002-0410-8

2 Tackla, M. (2003). Beautiful Minds?. *Dermatology Times*, 24(9), 78.

3 Lejour, M., & Lecocq, C. (1975). [Psychological implications of aesthetic surgery. A proposal of a study of 68 cases]. *Acta Chirurgica Belgica*, 74(1), 5-24.

4 Hern, J. J., Hamann, J. J., Tostevin, P. P., Rowe-Jones, J. J., & Hinton, A. A. (2002). Assessing psychological morbidity in patients with nasal deformity using the CORE® questionnaire. Clinical Otolaryngology & Allied Sciences, 27(5), 359-364.
5 Ibid.

6 Why People Want Plastic Surgery. (2005). *USA Today Magazine*, 134(2725), 2.
7 Ibid.

8 Suissa, A. (2008). Addiction to Cosmetic Surgery: Representations and Medicalization of the Body. *International Journal Of Mental Health & Addiction*, 6(4), 619-630.
9 Ibid.
10 Ibid.
11 Ibid.

12 Edelman, H. S. (1994). Why is Dolly Crying? An Analysis of Silicone Breast Implants in America as an Example of Medicalization. *Journal Of Popular Culture*, 28(3), 19-32.

13 Suissa, A. (2008). Addiction to Cosmetic Surgery: Representations and Medicalization of the Body. *International Journal Of Mental Health & Addiction*, 6(4), 619-630.
14 Ibid.

I did it. Now what?

CHAPTER FOUR

I have a limited recollection of the day of my surgery. I have no memory of being transported into the operating room. I remember a nurse talking to me before the surgery in my hospital room, but I don't remember receiving anesthesia, or seeing the surgeon that day.

I remember dressing in a hospital gown. I remember there was another girl my same age in my hospital room before I went to surgery. She knew who I was from school, but I didn't know her, and I don't remember her name or what she looked like. I don't know why she was in the hospital. I remember being embarrassed when she asked why I was there. I told her, but I really didn't want her to know the truth.

I was very groggy after the surgery. I remember waking up in the recovery room and my mom being there and asking how I was doing. I don't remember answering. I was heavily medicated. I was holding a new teddy bear my sister bought for me.

I didn't stay in the hospital overnight. It was a day procedure and I went home that afternoon. They gave me two blue bands of material that had elastic attached to it. I strapped one band around the bottom of my nose and the other one under my chin to catch any dripping blood from my incisions. I had an extra one for my new teddy bear. I didn't say much on the ride home. I ate ice chips and went to sleep. My face felt like a ton of bricks covered in cement.

At the time of my surgery, we were in the middle of a PCS—a change of duty station with the military. We were leaving Fort Stewart, Georgia and going to Fort Bragg, North Carolina. Almost no one outside of my immediate family, the staff at the hospital, and the unnamed girl in my hospital room, had any idea about my surgery.

I did tell one girl at my church that I was going to have cosmetic surgery. All she said was, "Why?" It really wasn't much of a conversation, and there wasn't any emotional connection between us. I didn't feel the support of a real friend. She had always kept me at arm's length. No amount of self-disclosure would change that.

I didn't have any other friends to tell. I didn't have any friends where I was going either. I didn't know anyone. According to my parents, it was better that no one knew about my surgery because people wouldn't understand, especially church people. It would be better if they didn't know. It was none of their business. My surgery was private and personal.

My life didn't change overnight after my surgery. My recovery process was both physical and emotional. I stayed inside for weeks, as if I were recovering from a long illness. The doctor had previously told me it would take at least a year before all of the swelling would be gone.

I did learn that my chin augmentation was greater than anticipated. The surgeon had planned to use a smaller sized chin implant, but he ended up using the largest implant he had. The idea was to bring balance to my face by extending my chin, instead of cutting away at my nose.

In the weeks immediately after my surgery, I had self-care procedures to tend to. There were stitches under my nose and chin. I can still picture the black thread weaving in and out of the puffy red areas of my face. I could feel the threads scratch the inside of my nose as I breathed.

My recovery wasn't as extensive as other people's because my surgery wasn't as invasive as it could have been. Only the lower part of the cartilage in my nose was removed. I've known other people who had to endure wound-packing high in their nasal cavity. I was glad I didn't have any packing to deal with. Wound-packing requires a lot of care, unpacking and repacking. It's quite a process every time the gauze needs changed.

In about a month, I was able to leave the house without strangers noticing my self-inflicted facial trauma. The military had already moved our household goods to North Carolina. I stayed with my sister at her apartment before I was ready to join my parents and brother in our new home.

I was a bit nervous about going to our new church in North Carolina. I had heard the church where we would be attending was more traditional and conservative than my family was. I felt my swelling hadn't gone down enough. I didn't want to risk anyone noticing the difference in my looks once the swelling went down further.

I was afraid the church people would judge me if they ever found out about my surgery. At the same time, all I really wanted was for them to accept me just as I was. I wanted them to know who I was, and what I had done to myself, yet to still love me. The risk was too great; I didn't tell anyone.

I was a senior in high school that year. I was attending a brand new school since we had just moved, and I felt as if I had a new lease on life. I had already completed most of the requirements to graduate, so I had an easy year. I only had one academic class—English, my favorite. My other classes included culinary arts, office assistant, and a class that oversaw the co-op early work-release program I was a part of.

Everyday, I left school early to go to work. My school placed me at my first job. I was a barista at a coffee shop on Fort Bragg. My parents bought me my first car, a used Toyota Camry. I was very happy and felt free for the first time in years. I don't know if I had ever felt so free.

Afterward

After my surgery, I wasn't free from pursuing perfectionism. I began to seek my ideal identity through increased religious performance and educational and career achievements. I didn't become addicted to cosmetic surgery, but I did sink deeper into perfectionism, and eventually became a workaholic.

The amazing thing about my imperfection (yes, ironically, perfectionism *is* an imperfection), is that God still saw incredible value in my life. It didn't matter that I thought I was worthless, or that I poured all of my energy into trying to be perfect. God saw beyond that. He saw my hurting heart.

The fact that I willingly continued to lay my life down at the altar of prayer allowed God to transform the negative qualities of my personality into an instrument for His grace. As long as I continue to allow Him room to work in my heart, He will take my life and make something better out of me than I could ever make out of myself.

Cosmetic surgery didn't change me, but God used it in my life as a part of His process. My life didn't radically change because of my surgery, but overtime God began to cut away negativity, hurt, and pain from my life. He began making me beautiful from the inside out, and I began to trust Him as I pursued His calling for my life.

I loved God, and continued to cultivate a relationship with Him despite my need for emotional healing. I felt close to the Lord. I read my Bible every day, and developed what I considered a strong prayer life. I had acknowledged a call to be a missionary when I was ten-years-old. I didn't know what all God had in store, but I was willing to go wherever He opened the door.

After graduating high school in 2001, I went on a mission trip to Kenya, Africa for ten days with a group of kids my age. I was seventeen and it was almost one year after my surgery. That mission trip was an influential experience I often think of.

We honestly didn't do much mission-work on our trip. We did form a choir and sang at an outdoor rally. A lot of what we did was sightsee and learn about the culture. I'll never forget going to the Masai Village and seeing the mud huts the women built. I loved going on safaris and seeing all of the beautiful animals. Their freedom was incredible, and trips to the zoo haven't been the same since then.

On that mission trip, I learned I was not cut out, or called, to be a missionary to a foreign country. I couldn't wait to get back to the United States. I missed my family and the safety of home. In transit back to the U.S., I and another girl were separated from our group. The airport gave our seats away to two Middle Eastern men and we were stuck in England with a nanny for five hours before the next flight out.

The mission trip was in June of 2001. I had planned to attend Bible College later that year, but the college closed for a year to relocate to a new campus. I stayed home and continued to work as a barista at the coffee shop on post.

I began to make close friends with some of the other young people at my church. I finally had a best friend. Her name was Miranda. I was so happy to have a friend who accepted me for who I was. I even told her about my cosmetic surgery, and she didn't judge me.

I went on my first date that year too. In fact, I had two boyfriends (at separate times) that year! I had never had a boyfriend before. It was a good year. I learned a lot about myself and I grew as a person. I continued to grow in my relationship with God.

I remember one night in particular I went to the prayer room at my church. It was a separately locked room that any member of the church who had a key could go to any time of the day or night to pray. I had been making a habit of going there to pray after work.

I began to pray for missionaries around the world, as I often did. There was a table in the church prayer room that had a notebook filled with missionaries' pictures and information on their countries. On the table was a small, soapstone egg I brought back from Kenya. It was painted like a globe. I brought it to the church and left it on the missions table after my trip.

I felt an odd feeling in the atmosphere that night. In an unusual act, I picked up the egg from the table and began to pray, holding "the world" in my hands. I felt an unusual heavy feeling that wouldn't leave. I didn't have the peace of God I usually felt when I prayed.

I had never done this before, nor since then, but for some reason I kissed that egg, the world. When I looked down, I had kissed America. At that moment, the power of God entered the prayer room in an almost tangible way, and broke off the heaviness I felt in my spirit. I immediately began to intercede, praying for my country. The intercession never left me that night. It was getting late and I had to work the next day, so I went home and continued to pray.

I woke up early and headed to work. It was September 11, 2001. I had no idea I would be making coffee for soldiers on Fort Bragg as terrorists hijacked four planes, and attacked the World Trade Center and Pentagon.

Everyone in the 82nd Airborne PX was quiet. We were all in shock. Soldiers gathered around TVs in the food court and stared in disbelief. Not only was our country under attack, all of our lives, which were a part of the military, could potentially be drastically affected.

Many of my coffee customers were members of the Special Forces. I remember two men in particular who left quickly that morning; I never saw them again. The news media didn't broadcast it, but a solider told me that Special Forces left for the Middle East within the hour of the first hijacking.

My father was still Active Duty Army. My boyfriend was too. Many of my friends and people I went to church with were about to go to war. My entire world caved in as those towers fell.

That night, the church opened its doors and we had a prayer meeting. My sister and I talked about how we felt and how afraid we were. We both sensed the military families were taking the news of 9/11 in a much more personal way than many of the civilian families were, though everyone was at a loss.

The rest of that year went by like a blur. I continued working. My dad retired from the Army in early 2002. I was set to head to Bible College that fall. I did go, but my heart was still in North Carolina. I kept in touch with friends and continually prayed for our military.

Several years later in the summer of 2010, one of the Army guys from our group of church friends was killed in Afghanistan. SSGT Christopher Todd Stout was one of the most sincere and God-loving people in our church. He was a member of the Army

Chorus, well-known for his soloist voice. He left behind a young wife and daughters. His death profoundly impacted everyone who knew him. It was so unexpected and tragic. I will never forget him singing the song "I Can Only Imagine."

You may wonder why I chose to share some of these stories. What do they have to do with cosmetic surgery? Well, nothing really, and I think that is the point. My life went forward after my choice to have surgery. Good things happened, and terrible things happened. The surgery really didn't have much of an impact on most of my life. A lot of other things—friendships, experiences, desires, a relationship with God—all of that took over, and I lived. I didn't change because of the surgery. I changed because I continued to live.

Psalm 90:12 KJV

Teach us to number our days,
that we may apply our hearts unto wisdom.

Questions for Reflection

- Have you ever had surgery of any kind before? What was your recovery process like?
- What are your plans and dreams for your life?
- What kind of people do you surround yourself with?
- Who is your best friend? What kind of character does he or she have?
- What is your life's purpose today?
- Do you feel God calling you to any other purpose?

Hidden Wounds

CHAPTER FIVE

> *"After their cosmetic surgery wounds have resolved, many people still need healing of their inner emotional wounds, which may be far more complex. [Many people achieve outer beauty, but remain lacking emotionally, without peace or contentment.]"*
> Dr. David H. McDaniel, M.D.[1]

We all go through painful circumstances in life. There are many times where I have been doubled over crying on the floor of my home after receiving terrible news about people I cared about. Pain is sacred; it changes us. Sometimes in our pain we make choices we wouldn't necessarily have made otherwise.

Can you name your pain? I can name mine—rejection. It's a big bundle of misunderstanding, abandonment, fear, neglect, being overlooked, interrupted, and not seriously listened to. At times, rejection overwhelms me. It's too big for me to figure out. It overtakes me and I'm left reeling.

When one of my triggers occurs, the pain of rejection immediately returns and kidnaps me away to a world of darkness. It doesn't seem to matter how much love I have in my life. I can even be cognizant of the people that love me, name them, acknowledge their love, and still be steeped in the unquenchable emotional pain of my current perceived rejection. I realize that the pain I feel is not totally dependent on an outside source, or lack of affection. The pain I feel is real, and it's coming from within me. It is like a type of PTSD that I cannot control.

A mentor once asked me to think about the one thing other people did that hurt me the most. I said it hurt me most when people don't listen to me.

"Well, it takes one to know one," he said. "Are you listening to yourself?"

He explained that we often don't like what we see in other people when they embody what we ourselves do. His statements and questions tugged at my heartstrings. He was speaking the truth. I hadn't been listening to myself. It wasn't long before I had a new understanding about my feelings of rejection.

Once I started listening to myself, I started acknowledging my own feelings and taking care of my heart. I started asking myself questions. *Was it possible that I was rejecting myself the whole time? Could the pain I feel when others reject me be intensified because it reinforces a deep-set belief I hold that I am not worthy of love and acceptance?*

From ten-years-old until the time of my surgery, I progressively spoke negativity to myself about myself. When I verbalized my thoughts, my parents tried to correct me. I was fifteen when my mother started forcing me to read self-help books, and I am so grateful she did.

Along with Bible reading and my relationship with God, reading books that taught me what was healthy and what was unhealthy was the start of my journey toward healing my damaged self-worth. One of the first books Mom gave me was Norman Vincent Peale's *The Power of Positive Thinking*. Another book she gave me was *The Seven Habits of Highly Effective Teens*, by Sean Covey.

In this chapter, I'm going to tell the story of what happened in the years prior to my surgery. I was sixteen-years-old, almost seventeen, when I chose cosmetic surgery. I hadn't done a lot of introspection at that point in my life. I was simply surviving. I didn't have the emotional skills or strength to do anything else.

Inner Damage

The five years prior to my surgery were difficult years for me. It started when I was in 7th grade. I guess that's a typical time for struggles to begin. Middle school is no joke. We lived in a small town about thirty minutes outside of Fort Hood, Texas.

That year was the first year I responded to the calling I felt in my heart to be a missionary. I wasn't loud about it, but I did try. I shared a Bible study video with all of my teachers, and several responded positively. Only one—my science teacher—refused to watch the video.

I asked for permission to put invitational fliers into the teacher's boxes in the main office, inviting all the teachers in the whole public school to attend a special revival at my church. The office approved my request, and two teachers from the school came to the revival.

Later that year, my science teacher told our class the Bible was full of fables. I told my mom, who in-turn complained to the principal. The teacher was reprimanded, and later pulled me into her walk-in storage closet, sternly letting me know her displeasure.

"If you have a problem with something I say, you need to come to me first," she said. As if she was approachable. She made the rest of the year quite difficult for me.

I also started to experience bullying from older kids. They would make fun of the way I dressed, calling me a pilgrim. The truth was, I really had no sense of fashion whatsoever, and I dressed from the old-lady's petite department at the local mall. If you can imagine what a typical "home-school kid" might have dressed like in the 90s, I more than likely looked worse. Of course, I went to public school the whole time. Still, I always minded my own business, and I certainly didn't deserve the name-calling.

We moved to Virginia the summer before I started 8th grade. I was okay with moving. It was a new adventure, but I was going to miss our house and the few friends I had. The teachers at my new school treated all of us as if we were horrible children who didn't know how to behave. Most of the kids in my classes didn't know how to behave. It was a challenging year filled with a lot of screaming adults.

The most difficult part of 8th grade was gym class. The first week of school my male gym teacher handed me a pair of super-short red shorts, and told me I had to wear them and a white tee-shirt to his class. It was the school's dress code for gym class, he said.

I already mentioned my fashion sense, but the way I dressed also had to do with my Christian beliefs. Since I'm writing a book about my experience with cosmetic surgery, you may find it somewhat controversial to know exactly how conservative my family was. I wore dresses all of the time, and never cut my hair. I had never worn shorts in public and I certainly wasn't about to start in 8th grade during the height of my insecurities in that awkward puberty stage.

I explained my position to my gym teacher.

He glared at me. "I've researched your religion and not wearing shorts isn't a part of it. Go to the principal's office," he barked at me. He didn't even know what religion I was.

As I walked toward the door he changed his mind. "Go to the counselor's office instead," he yelled.

We ended up having a huge meeting with myself, my mom, my gym teacher, and another coach at the school. My mother patiently explained our church's dress code and the reasoning behind not showing the shape of our legs or skin above the knee.

"I think you will feel more comfortable in the other gym class," the coach said to me at the meeting. In reality, I think he was going to be more comfortable with me out of his sight. We all agreed to switch my class, but we didn't discuss any further details about the class I was moving to.

When I went to my new gym class the next day, it was the "Special Education" class. There were several students there with severe mental disabilities and birth defects, as well as a group of deaf students. I had never been around people with special needs before. This was back in the late 90s prior to their inclusion into regular classrooms.

To be honest, I was shocked when I entered the room. I had no idea I was not swapping into another regular gym class. I remember one student with severe mental issues rolling around on the floor, screaming. Another would stare at me, drool, and smile.

I now have compassion in my heart for students and people with disabilities, but at that time I was afraid. As an 8th grader, I was treated as if I too had a mental or physical disability. I was not used as a helper, or treated differently than the other students.

There was no interaction between the "regular" kids and the "special" kids. Our gym activities took place on the back side of the school, in the small gym where no one would see us. The problem was, they paraded our "special" class in a line through the school to get where we were going, as if we were in elementary school. The other middle schoolers (who are very cruel) noticed that I was in the "special" class. I was supposed to sit with my new class at lunch, but thankfully my new coach let me sit with a friend from another class instead.

It was a difficult year. A girl from one of my other classes asked me if there was something wrong with my legs, and if that is why I wore skirts and was in the special class. I didn't know what to say. I didn't explain. I just said, "No." I caved in on myself emotionally that year. My anxiety was at an all-time high. I believe it was also my first experience with depression. At that time, I had never heard about anxiety and depression, and I certainly couldn't name my feelings.

The daily time I spent excluded from the regular gym class due to my religious preference to wear skirts gnawed at me. I felt out of place, rejected, and unwanted. I knew I was perfectly capable of running laps and playing sports in a full skirt or culottes, but that first coach wouldn't consider it. The isolation I experienced during gym class did a lot of damage to my already fragile 13-year-old self-esteem.

I remember being in the locker room crying one day. One of the deaf students saw me crying and tried to comfort me, but she and I couldn't communicate, and the last thing I wanted was attention. She found the coach and brought her to me.

"Do you want to go back into the other class?" The coach asked.

"No. I can't go back to his class," I said with my head down. I couldn't look my new coach in the eyes. I felt so low. I kept thinking of the coach that didn't want me. I would rather be in a class where I didn't belong, and was made fun of by other kids, than to be in a class where the teacher didn't want me. I didn't want to experience bullying from the coach like I had experienced from my science teacher the year before.

Despite my 8th grade bout with depression and anxiety, the experience fueled me to prove to the world that I was smart and capable. But first I had to know it for myself, and that would take many years.

I did have two friends in 8th grade. One was Elizabeth, who was an agnostic, and the other was Julia, an atheist Russian immigrant. We would play in the creek and ravines that ran through our neighborhood, and hang out at each other's houses. I remember

Julia's family was very open about not believing in God. I found it funny that they had a Christmas tree with Santa Clause ornaments all over it. They called it their "New Year's Tree."

We lived in Virginia for one year, and moved the next summer to Silver Spring, Maryland on other side of Washington D.C. I missed my friends, but would not miss my school. In 9th grade, at another new school, I faced an entirely new challenge—racial prejudice. JKF High School was about 95 percent African American, 3 percent Asian, and 2 percent white.

Midway into the year, two African American girls chased me down a hallway and into a bathroom because they didn't like me. I was the only white girl in our cooking class. They started taunting me and backed me up against the far wall of the bathroom. I know they would have beat me up if the janitor hadn't come in and stopped them.

As the janitor stood between me and the girls, I ran out of the bathroom, down the stairwell and straight to the counselor's office. I can still hear those girls laughing as I ran away. The African American counselor told me I needed to get over it because I was "privileged." My heart was wounded in yet another way—that counselor was just one more adult who didn't take the time to protect or love me.

The rest of that school year was filled with a lot of anxiety. I hated riding the bus and would often be "late" and miss it. We rode three to a seat, those of us in the aisle had to hang on for dear life. To top it off, our bus driver played loud rap music, which I hated.

There were constant fights at the school. Every day during my algebra class, someone would pull the fire alarm and we would all have to go outside for the rest of the class. Later that year, an older student at our school was on the news for murder. He fled the country, going to Israel where he had citizenship. It seemed like there was no end to the news of violence and fear attached to that school.

I did make a couple of friends that year. One was a kind and quiet girl named Ravneet. She was a Sikh, a follower of Sikhism—a monotheistic Indian religion. We shared several common values. I remember when Ravneet came up to me at school. She asked me about my hair because it was so long. She also didn't cut her hair. She invited me to her house. I learned that no one in their family cut their hair, and I had the opportunity to watch her mom and sister help her dad roll up his hair into a turban.

Another friend was Latonya. She had beautiful long braids and lived in the projects near the school. We were in gym class together. I remember her randomly telling me that she had just learned about abstinence from the Young Life group she was a part of. She had never heard of it before.

The next summer we moved to a small Southern town in Georgia. We were there for my 10th and 11th grade years. I went to an almost entirely white school in the old South. It was a completely different culture than Maryland where there were a lot of different races and religions.

I finally met my first two Christian friends since leaving Texas. I had always been a naturally quiet person, so making friends didn't come easily for me, especially with all of the moving around and the bullying I faced. I thought having Christian friends would be a great experience. It was the first time I had friends I felt I could share my faith with.

It wasn't long before what I thought was an answer to my prayers—my two new Christian friends—became another source of rejection and pain. The girls were of a different Christian denomination than I was, and someone at their church counseled them that my church was full of the devil. They kicked me out of their Bible study, and told me to stay away from them. It was as if they couldn't wrap their minds around me because I wasn't just like them. I was an outsider, and they made sure it stayed that way.

I didn't understand. Why did it matter how I dressed or that my denomination had a different name than theirs did? I loved Jesus with all of my heart. I never disrespected their church. Why would they stop being my friends because I was different? I was a good person.

After that, I didn't try anymore. I began drifting into more and more isolation. I increased my exercise, decreased my eating, and watched a lot of old black and white musicals. I wanted to believe good times existed, and I wanted to push forward, but there was still such hurt inside. All I wanted was to be accepted for who I was. I had to be strong and make it through the next year and half before I could move again.

I didn't make any more friends after those girls rejected me. I isolated and quietly entertained myself. I didn't know it at the time, but looking back, I can see I was struggling with very strong anxiety and depression. I was angry, but instead of exploding out on everyone else, I imploded in on myself and became more and more negative toward my self-image. I believed the rejection of others meant something was wrong with me.

I didn't share my feelings. I didn't know how to put my struggle into words. It was, and often still is, difficult for me to verbally express my feelings. It's not something my family does. It's much easier for me to write down my feelings than to verbalize them.

My parents didn't know what to do to help me. Out of frustration, my mom started making me read the self-help books. My parents knew I wasn't happy with my nose; it was about the only thing I complained about. My dad told me he had a friend who was a plastic surgeon. He said if I wanted cosmetic surgery, his friend would do it for me. I think Dad thought it would make me happy to change my looks.

I hadn't considered cosmetic surgery before my dad brought it up. I didn't know much about it. I didn't know anything really. But I knew I was in pain and I thought it was my fault because I wasn't good enough. Anything I could do to improve myself, I was willing to do it. If it would help me feel better about myself, and if I didn't have to compromise what I believed, I would go for it.

It was very important to me to have the approval of the people around me. I wanted my parents, my church, my teachers and my peers to accept me. If having a smaller nose would help me love myself more so I could stop hating myself and start living, I would do it.

I prayed about the decision. I knew something had to change. I realized I was not in a good place internally, and I didn't know what else to do to help myself. It was an opportunity and I took it.

It wasn't long after the surgery that I knew within my heart and soul that cosmetic surgery was not the answer to my problems. It didn't bring me happiness or transform me into a popular girl. I had to learn how to make conversation. I had to learn to function while being different and unknown.

Difficulties Communicating

Communication facilitates our relationships. When we have trouble communicating, our relationships suffer. When contemplating undergoing a cosmetic procedure, I think it's important to consider the impact it may have on non-verbal communication, particularly if the surgery is on the face.

Humans communicate emotion through facial expressions. If a cosmetic procedure alters the face, it could potentially interfere with non-verbal communication. No doubt, every procedure has a varied physical effect. Some procedures may only have a temporary effect, while others may leave permanent nerve damage.

Botox, for example, eliminates wrinkles in the skin by blocking nerve signals to the muscle.[2] The muscles freeze, paralyzing injected areas for a period of months. Living with paralyzed facial muscles can increase miscommunication.

The lack of ability to express ourselves non-verbally may also hinder brain circuits coordinating emotion.[3] Studies show emotions intensify depending on the facial expressions presented.[4] For example, you may be unhappy at work, but if you choose to smile, your emotions are likely to follow. We show sensitivity to others by reading and mimicking facial expressions as we interact with those around us. Some cosmetic procedures may actually work against non-verbal communication.[5]

Though my surgery did not impact my ability to non-verbally express my emotions, I still feel the lasting physical effect of my choice. Over fifteen years later, I still feel facial discomfort and experience numbness in my lips and chin in cold weather and under stress. Though I've grown accustom to it, I always feel a tightness in my face that wasn't there before. I have some nerve damage. The risk of permanent damage, even something minor like I experience, is important to consider when making a decision about elective cosmetic surgery.

Born Again

In my research, I read a story about a woman who turned to cosmetic surgery after her husband left their long-time marriage. She wanted a new life, and to start over fresh. She called her cosmetic surgery journey a "born-again" experience.[6] She was willing to do anything for the feeling of acceptance. For her, cosmetic surgery wasn't about finding a new husband, it was just about obtaining the attentions, even momentarily, of any man. She was thwarting the pain of rejection by chasing new experiences that affirmed her in the face of her husband's rejection.

There is only one way to be born again, and its through the water and the Spirit (John 3:5). There isn't a surgery in the world that will take away inner pain or make you into a new person. Only the transforming power of the Holy Spirit can give you new life—and not just new life, but eternal life.

I've learned that even with the power of God clearly moving in my life, I still have issues and problems to deal with. God can use me in the condition I am in, but that doesn't spare me from life's hurt. Life still happens to us all, even after finding salvation, and moving forward in God's plan for our lives.

Even with God's Spirit overflowing in my life as He does, this human body won't walk on streets of gold—regardless of outward beauty, dress codes, or cosmetic alterations. It's my soul God saves, not my flesh. He renews my spirit and takes me to new heights in His love, but I still feel the ups and downs of this world within my emotions.

A couple of years ago I fell off of one step as I was packing my storage unit to move back in with my parents after I experienced a job layoff. I twisted my foot and ankle and was in a lot of pain. I had never sprained or broken anything in my life and I had no idea how severe my injury was. I went to a walk-in clinic and they did an x-ray. They said it was a bad sprain.

After that, I rested for several weeks, trying to stay off of my ankle. I had a lot of time to pray. During one of my prayer times, the Lord quietly spoke to my heart. *"You have no idea how broken you are. There is so much more to life that you haven't experienced."*

Six weeks after my accident, I learned I had broken my right talus bone, the bone beneath all of the other bones that make up the ankle. The talus bone is apparently the most difficult bone in the body to break. Normally, people break it snowboarding. It only took me falling off of one step. I endured a delayed healing. It was 8 months before I was able to put on a pair of high heels again. I still have some residual pain from the broken ankle.

A big part of the delay in healing was that I didn't stop walking like I should have. I kept putting pressure on myself to get better. I didn't know my ankle was broken, but I did know it hurt. Still, I pushed myself. Healing takes time, but I didn't want to wait.

Looking back, my heart was very wounded when I made the choice for cosmetic surgery. I really didn't have a lot of time for my heart to heal after every military move we made, the losses associated with that, and the personal rejection I kept experiencing. I had a lot of soul-wounds in the years after my surgery as well. Those stories are for another book.

At the time of my surgery, my heart was broken, and I kept running into hurt and pain that injured me over and over again. I didn't rest in God's love or allow Him to mend me back together again. I kept pushing myself to do more, and be better. It took a broken bone to force me to stop and take some time for my heart to heal over some of these very old wounds.

Just a few months after I broke my ankle, the Lord began leading me to write this book. I knew the timing was right. I wanted to move on to other projects and other dreams, but it was as if I had to write this book first. I can see why now. There was so much I needed to learn about myself and so much I needed to sort through from long ago. All of the hurt from back then kept being pushed down deeper and deeper through the years, buried under more hurt. But it was all still there under the surface.

While in Bible College in 2004, the Lord led me to Isaiah Chapter 54. It became one of my favorite chapters in the Bible. The entire chapter spoke to me in a variety of ways, but verses 11 and 12 stood out to me the most.

> *O thou afflicted, tossed with tempest, and not comforted, behold, I will lay thy stones with fair colours, and lay thy foundations with sapphires. And I will make thy windows of agates, and thy gates of carbuncles, and all thy borders of pleasant stones.*

After all of the storms of my life, through all of the times I seemed to lack comfort, God gave me a promise that He would build stability and beauty into my life. As I look back over it all, I am amazed at the work He has done and continues to do.

And now, He's using my story to speak into your life these same promises. He's not finished building beauty into your life. There may be tempests, but He is the Storm-Calmer. There may be a lack of boundaries, but He is the Builder of the wall and gate. There may be hidden wounds of the heart, but He is the best Surgeon there is. He makes all things beautiful in His time (Ecclesiastes 3:11).

Jeremiah 17:14 KJV

Heal me, O LORD, and I shall be healed; save me, and I shall be saved: for thou art my praise.

Questions for Reflection

- How do you talk to yourself about yourself? If your best friend talked to you the way you talk to you, would you stay in the relationship?
- Do you have any brokenness you have not yet healed from? Do you have hidden wounds that need tending to?
- Are you experiencing anxiety or depression?
- Are you considering cosmetic surgery as a way to start over after a major loss?
- What is your relationship with God like? Are you open to receiving the beauty God wants to create in you?

Endnotes

1. Tackla, M. (2003). Beautiful Minds?. *Dermatology Times*, *24*(9), 78.

2. Wheatley, M. (2012). Healthy Beauty, Cosmetic Treatments, Botox. www.*WebMD.com/beauty/botox/cosmetic-procedures-botox*.

3. Bower, B. (2010). Effects of Botox go beyond the face. *Science News*, *178*(3), 8.
4. Ibid.
5. Ibid.

6. Kinnunen, T. (2010). 'A second youth': Pursuing happiness and respectability through cosmetic surgery in Finland. *Sociology Of Health & Illness*, *32*(2), 258-271.

The Quest

CHAPTER SIX

"All too often, the world we live in sends the message that we have to consume things to be happy, that we can buy beauty and happiness. Sometimes, people get confused by this and it is obvious during [surgery] consultation..."
Dr. McDaniel, Dermatologic Cosmetic Surgeon[1]

What is your quest in life? What do you think will make you happy? Will plastic surgery help you obtain your goal? In this chapter, I will speculate on four common reasons for pursuing happiness through cosmetic surgery: beauty, youthfulness, love, and ideal identity.

The Quest for Beauty

1 Peter 3:3-4 The Message

What matters is not your outer appearance—the styling of your hair, the jewelry you wear, the cut of your clothes—but your inner disposition. Cultivate inner beauty, the gentle, gracious kind that God delights in.

Beauty is power. I've heard it my entire life. The statement is the first half of a line by Charles Reade, a writer from the 1800s. The quote in full is: "Beauty is power; a smile is its sword." Why is beauty powerful? I think beauty is powerful because it can capture the attention and hearts of the people around us. Beauty can influence, and influence is powerful.

Beauty reflects power to me. Beauty and order motivate me to clean and decorate my house, to create a fun birthday cake for someone I love, and to do my best to present beauty to the world in every work of art I create. My value of beauty also gives me an appreciation for everything from architecture, to the wildflowers alongside the road.

I am a visual person in the way I learn, the way I communicate, and the way I connect to the world around me. When I see the vulnerability of a homeless person on the street, I feel compassion. When I see the joyful expressions on the faces of children as they play, I feel happy. As a visual person, when the world around me is organized and beautiful, my inner life seems to line up and become beautiful as well. Making something beautiful gives me a sense of control in my ever-changing world.

As a young adult, I projected my own visual approach to life onto other people. Because beauty motivated me and I appreciated it so much, I assumed others viewed the world the same way I did. In high school, outward appearance seemed connected to social acceptance, and that confirmed my belief in the power of beauty.

As a young person struggling to find my place, I desired one thing: to belong. I bought into the idea that social acceptance was based on the outward appearance of confidence. If I could exude confidence, then perhaps my peers would accept me, I thought. I watched people who were confident. They all seemed so beautiful and happy. As a visual person, I began pursuing confidence from the outside in, conforming to fashion and trends. I was on a quest for beauty.

As a teenager, after failing to successfully enter a social group during 10th and 11th grade in Georgia, I began comparing myself to other girls my age. After that one particularly harsh rejection experience, instead of holding my peers responsible for the way they treated me, I became critical toward myself. I convinced myself I was less than they required.

A year later, I turned to cosmetic surgery in order to correct what I believed was unacceptable. I was not focused on God's acceptance of me just as I was. Instead, I was willing to change everything about myself in order to gain the acceptance of my peers.

At some point I had to ask myself the question, how much will I allow what others think of me to control me? Why did I place such value on the opinion of others?

Galatians 1:10 ESV

For am I now seeking the approval of man, or of God?
Or am I trying to please man? If I were still trying to please man,
I would not be a servant of Christ.

There is a danger in judging ourselves and others based on outward appearance. We certainly cannot know another person by looking at them. We can't determine the state of their inner wholeness, their relationship with God, or their health as person based on the way they look.

There are a lot of people who are beautiful, and know how to act and present themselves in a socially acceptable way, but privately they behave in harmful and unhealthy ways. That's why when we truly get to know someone, they either become more attractive, or more unattractive than we originally thought.

Some of the most amazing and inspiring people I've met aren't physically attractive. Some of them have birth defects or injuries that damaged them. But these same people have a depth of soul that shines beyond the outside so much that they are the most beautiful people I've ever met.

In contrast, I've met some people who feel the world owes them because they were born with a defect. Others use their injuries to manipulate people into feeling sorry for them, so they can get their way. The same is true for some naturally beautiful people. Some of them act entitled and others use their beauty to manipulate.

True beauty is not a result of cosmetic surgery. It's a matter of the heart. Whether or not you choose surgery doesn't matter as much as the condition of your heart. Who you are will shine regardless of what you look like. When we seek to mature and to glorify God in and through our bodies, our inner beauty will shine brighter than the most beautiful look we could ever hope to attain.

1 Samuel 16:7 KJV

The Lord seeth not as man seeth; for man looketh on the outward appearance, but the Lord looketh on the heart.

The Quest for Youthfulness

Proverbs 31:30 NKJV

Charm is deceitful and beauty is passing, but a woman who fears the Lord, she shall be praised.

I watched a makeover reality TV show in which a woman in her 70s underwent multiple cosmetic surgeries. She looked like a different woman by the time the makeover crew finished with her, and, yes, she was beautiful.

The part of the show that I remember the most was the very end. The reality host was following up with the woman after several weeks of recovery from all the surgery. During the last several seconds of the last episode, the "new" woman stood at her front door as the camera crew filmed her from a distance.

It was the look in the woman's face and eyes that I remember the most. I watched her standing there, looking out from within her changed body. She was smiling, but the smile was tense. I could see reality dawning on her face. Inside she was the same woman, but she had lost a part of herself through the makeover. She had lost the smile lines it took years to make. She had lost the wrinkle lines in her forehead from all the times she had worried about the people she loved.

Was what I saw a look of masked disappointment, or was it the reality of life in plastic, possible nerve damage, or loss of facial expression? Did she lose a sense of connection with her older friends who still looked their age? I can only imagine how I would feel if I were that woman.

I've heard some older women gossiping about others who have had "work" done. Their jealous spirits can be quite tormenting. Among the World War II generation, attitudes about cosmetic plastic surgery are often negative.[2] The social pressure against plastic surgery leaves many older patients feeling as if they cannot openly talk about their surgery to their peers without judgment.

Western culture glamorizes youth. It seems everyone wants to look young. To be young is to be full of life, health, energy, and happiness. Thankfully, due to advances in medical care, people are living longer and staying healthier than in previous generations. Many people want to enjoy their bodies as long as they can, and that may mean turning to plastic surgery as a way to recover youthfulness and to obtain a sense of happiness.

The physical transformation of cosmetic surgery can bring a renewed sense of youth and seemingly prevent aging. Many older cosmetic surgery patients expressed they had self-actualized in middle-age. That means middle-age was the first time in their life they truly saw their own worth and fully lived out their potential. These older patients came to think of themselves as middle-aged and no longer recognized themselves in the mirror. They used plastic surgery as a way of becoming "themselves" again.[3]

Patients who suffer from reduced self-image due to aging are considered good candidates for plastic surgery.[5] In a culture that idealizes youth, cosmetic surgery can become the gateway to holding onto relationships, jobs, and a feeling of vitality and purpose within the mainstream community. When middle-aged or older people go under the knife for cosmetic reasons, they often associate it with their quality of life.[6]

Some people choose plastic surgery as a way of "positive aging" or defying the aging process by staying healthy, happy, and looking youthful. One woman said she was taking responsibility for keeping up her appearance as she aged by undergoing plastic surgery. Many older women said they weren't trying to hide their age with cosmetic surgery, but rather they wanted to look good for their age.[7]

A 76-year old woman explained her choice to have eyelid surgery, a face-lift, and liposuction as it related to her active lifestyle. She said she could never be the type of person to sit at home knitting in her rocking chair. She didn't want to look like she was 100 years old; instead she wanted to look "good" as she participated in activities.[8]

I believe it is important that we foster an appreciation and respect for aging. Is it possible for us to see beauty in a wrinkled face? I hope so! If not, we may find our culture at greater risk of ageism and becoming an anti-aging society. At the worst, our culture could begin moving toward senicide (suicide of elderly) or geronticide (killing of the elderly) if we continue to devalue aging.

Life is precious and sacred. One of the best ways we can honor our elders is to honor aging and all that comes with it. If our culture views the aging process as a disease or deformity, what will my generation's quality of life be like in the sunset years?

I am currently in my early thirties. At this point in my life, I have no desire to ever have plastic surgery again. What if, as I grow older, I begin to miss the way I looked when I was younger? If I have the money, will I choose to spend it on a face-lift?

I hope my answer is no, but I can't say now what I'll choose later. I'll be a different woman then. I can't promise that I'll never have plastic surgery again. I have no idea what the future holds, or what I will experience throughout my life.

All I know is that I want to be a woman who pleases God. I want to care for the world around me, love the people I have in my life, and take care of those I can help. I want to age with grace and be a living example of a true Christian that generations after me can follow. As I age, I want my sense of self-worth to flourish, not based on the way I look, but based on God's value of me.

I hope I would take the money I would spend on surgery and put it toward some kind of humanitarian mission. Instead of spending the money on myself, what if I paid for plastic surgery for children in a third world country who are suffering from a birth defect or abnormality that would prevent them from ever being able to support themselves or their family? These are the questions I'm asking myself now so that I can have a vision of the type of woman I want to be in the future.

I can't help but think of my Papaw who passed away earlier this year at the age of 89. He was here in our home when he died. How precious he was to me. His white hair, his frail frame, his blue eyes. I loved him, and still do. There is not a thing I would change about the way he looked.

I loved his wrinkles. I loved his smile. I loved his unchecked personality. His character was so beautifully expressed through his aged body. He lived his life to the fullest, and it was not at all based on the way he looked.

Isaiah 46:4 NIV

Even to your old age and gray hairs I am he, I am he who will sustain you. I have made you and I will carry you; I will sustain you and I will rescue you.

The Quest for Love

"Let someone love you just the way you are – as flawed as you might be, as unattractive as you sometimes feel, and as unaccomplished as you think you are. To believe that you must hide all the parts of you that are broken, out of fear that someone else is incapable of loving what is less than perfect, is to believe that sunlight is incapable of entering a broken window and illuminating a dark room." -Marc Chernoff

Love. What would you be willing to do, give, or trade for love? Many trade purity and loyalty to secure the love of another person. Others use money to capture attention and buy affection. Some use plastic surgery as a way to reach cultural beauty ideals in order to secure the attention, admiration, and love of another person.

We will sacrifice a lot to find and keep love. What if accepting your flaws and learning to feel comfortable in your body would open the door to love? Would you be willing to go there? Would you be willing to live imperfectly and embrace your flaws if *that* were the cost for love?

Our American ideas about love can be a bit skewed at times. Some of us believe love is all about a good feeling and a rush of hormones. Others over-give themselves to relationships and endure all types of abuse in the name of love.

I'm learning that love is somewhere in the middle of the two extremes. Love can be wonderful and it can also painful, which is what makes it so confusing. There's nothing greater than feeling close to someone, and there is no greater pain than watching someone you love go through a difficult time and not be able to do anything about it.

Regardless of the people in life who love us, it is our perception of ourselves that predicates how much love we perceive is in our lives. If we believe we are unworthy of love, then we will reject love no matter how much is available to us. If we believe we are worthy of love, then we will accept love no matter how undeserving the world says we are.

The same goes for how much love we give. If we believe we have love to give, we will give it to those around us. If we believe we are running on empty and unable to give to others, we will not freely give love to the people in our lives. How much love do you have available to give to others?

In Mark 12:31, the Bible tells us to love our neighbors as we love ourselves. It seems like that verse didn't take into consideration that some people do not love themselves. Some people hate themselves so very much. They do not feel worthy of love and cannot accept it from others. They do not have love inside of them to offer to the people around them.

In the quest for love, which we all undoubtedly pursue, there is only one thing for us to remember. God's love is available for us to receive, and when we receive it, we will overflow with love for others. Have you tapped into God's abundant and unconditional love?

Cosmetic surgery will never produce love in our lives. Only we can choose to love and be loved, and that choice must be separate from a choice about surgery. A person who loves us will never ask or demand for us to change our bodies and risk our lives by undergoing cosmetic surgery. If a person we love suggests we put ourselves through a physically traumatic procedure such as cosmetic surgery, it's time to start asking some hard questions about the health of the relationship.

I once heard the story of a plastic surgeon who married a woman he supposedly loved. He preformed surgery after surgery on the woman to bring her looks up to his personal standard of beauty.

He said he loved her soul, but not her body. How is that possible? He wanted to conform her to his ideal image of a woman. He risked her life over and over, for his own selfishness.

In another story, a man divorced his wife after he deemed their children were ugly. He found out after the birth of his children that his wife had previously undergone multiple cosmetic surgeries. He claimed she lied to him by keeping her surgeries a secret. He claimed she owed him because their children were "ugly."

How can a man call himself a man if he would divorce his wife and leave his children because he thinks they are ugly? He had a sick kind of selfishness and was psychologically abusive as he rejected the people who needed his love the most. Selfishness is not love at all.

A person who loves you will not ask you to go out of your way, to go through pain to enhance their own pleasure. Radically the opposite, a person who loves you will make themselves uncomfortable, and be willing to hurt for you. They will endure difficult times with you and support you to the best of their ability.

True love is not dependent on what we look like or how cool our personality is. True love cannot be bought or earned.

1 Corinthians 13:4-8 ESV

Love is patient and kind; love does not envy or boast; it is not arrogant or rude. It does not insist on its own way; it is not irritable or resentful; it does not rejoice at wrongdoing, but rejoices with the truth. Love bears all things, believes all things, hopes all things, endures all things. Love never ends.

The Quest for Ideal Identity

2 Corinthians 10:12 ESV

Not that we dare to classify or compare ourselves with some of those who are commending themselves. But when they measure themselves by one another and compare themselves with one another, they are without understanding.

Do you have an image in your mind of an ideal person? What does that person look like? Maybe it is someone you know. Maybe it is someone you respect—a mentor or a leader you admire. Does watching that person's life inspire you to be a better person and to improve various aspects about yourself? You may not have an actual person you can name, but is there an ideal in your mind that you compare yourself to?

I picked up a brochure from a plastic surgery center near where I live. Their slogan is: "More beautiful . . . More youthful . . . More you." Aesthetic surgeons often legitimize cutting a functioning body by arguing they are producing psychological benefits.[9] As one writer reported: "[Cosmetic surgery] is an exercise of power primarily related to identity. Having plastic surgery serves to reproduce the normal, the better than normal, and the best."[10] But where is the statistical evidence?

When I chose cosmetic surgery, I had an ideal image in my mind of who I wanted to be. My ideal image went beyond outward appearance—it also included character, spirituality, and social status. I wanted to become my own ideal. I was not comfortable with my body, or honest about my character flaws. I worked hard to hide my issues from other people, but I couldn't hide the reality from myself. I was obsessed with my imperfections and my quest to obtain my own ideal identity.

There are many women today who use cosmetic surgery to try to transform their bodies to obtain an ideal image. Some women even try to transform their bodies into their husband's ideal image in order to gain his attention and affection. I have to question the authenticity of love and intimacy in relationships where one partner constantly changes his or herself—bodily or behaviorally—in order to please the other partner and obtain relational and emotional commitment.

Saint-Hilaire wrote that people often enhance their bodies in order to actualize their own identity.[11] That means, people who alter their bodies with cosmetic surgery are exerting power over their own bodies to transform themselves into the image they want for themselves. In order to enter into their full and complete identity, they must transform into their own idol.

Presenting another view, author Mario Gonzalez-Ulloa argued that changing the external appearance restores inner light, just as an inner spiritual change brings an external glow. The idea that changing the outside can change the inside is an "outside-in" mentality.[12]

These opposing ideas remind me of Julian Rotter's 1954 theory of *locus of control*. When a person has an internal locus of control, they believe they are internally responsible for their thoughts, actions, behaviors, and the direction of their life. They are in control of their own responses to life.

A person with an external locus of control believes people, life experiences, and the world around them control their emotional state, reactions, decisions, and ultimately what happens to them. They do not take responsibility for their emotional reactions, or internal state. They constantly look to others to validate them.

I believe that people who take personal responsibility for their emotions (internal locus of control) who choose to have a cosmetic procedure are more in line with Saint-Hilaire's view of self-actualization. On the other hand, I think people who believe the world around them controls their emotions (external locus of control), would tend to believe cosmetic surgery will change the inside, as Gonzalez-Ulloa suggested.

When I was sixteen, I had an external locus of control. Several years later, I learned about Rotter's theory. The knowledge of the theory challenged me to start consciously taking responsibility for my internal state.

From my personal experience, I do not believe changing the outside ever changes the inside. If changing the outside changed the inside, we could easily free people from additions, mental illness, and character defects by changing their clothes and hairstyles. Real change must come from within the mind and patterns of self-talk.

A makeover may inspire a person to see they are not trapped in their current identity and may give them the motivation to improve their level of self-respect. But if their beliefs remain the same, a made-over person will eventually revert to negative self-talk and old grooming habits, which accurately reflect their true beliefs about themselves.

Cosmetic surgery was a part of my journey toward accepting my flaws and letting go of my quest for an ideal identity. I needed the experience to help me see beyond myself. The bodily pain I experienced post-op was intense; after all, I had just put myself through major physical trauma. The physical pain took my mind off of my inner pain for a while, and helped me readjust my perspective of life. Cosmetic surgery didn't change the way I felt about myself, but the experience gave me a reality check about my own emotional health.

During the months of waiting for my facial swelling to go down, I experienced the rock-bottom realization of where my self-talk had taken me. I knew I didn't want to continue in the same patterns. I didn't have the strength to change myself, and I knew it. I turned to God and His loving power to lift me from the self-defeating beliefs I held.

Cosmetic surgery did not transform me into my ideal identity. Instead, it helped me to realize I'm a flawed human who will never be perfect, and that is okay. The love, comfort and acceptance of Christ began to flood my heart. I began to experience greater dependency on God and realized He loved me just for who I was. I learned how to accept and appreciate my body and its flaws. I adjusted my patterns of thought and began the transition to a new, positive, and grace-filled identity.

Questions for Reflection

- What motivates you toward cosmetic surgery? Is it beauty, youthfulness, love, or ideal identity?
- How much do you value beauty?
- Is your interpretation of beauty based on popular culture?
- Is your self-worth healthy enough to carry you through the aging process?
- Do you think you will pursue cosmetic surgery as you age?
- What kind of older person do you want to be?
- What do you want your life to be about?
- What do you want to spend your money on?
- Do you love your imperfections?
- Do you love the imperfections you see in the people around you?
- Do you base your identity on an internal or external locus of control? In other words, do you take personal responsibility for your emotions, or do you believe other people and circumstances control your internal experience?
- Do you believe changing your body will automatically change your inner experience of life?

Endnotes

1   Tackla, M. (2003). Beautiful Minds?. *Dermatology Times*, 24(9), 78.

2   Kinnunen, T. (2010). 'A second youth': Pursuing happiness and respectability through cosmetic surgery in Finland. *Sociology Of Health & Illness*, 32(2), 258-271.

3   Kinnunen, T. (2010). 'A second youth': Pursuing happiness and respectability through cosmetic surgery in Finland. *Sociology Of Health & Illness*, 32(2), 258-271.

4   American Society of Plastic Surgeons. PlasticSurgery.org. 2013.

5   Tackla, M. (2003). Beautiful Minds?. *Dermatology Times*, 24(9), 78.

6   Kinnunen, T. (2010). 'A second youth': Pursuing happiness and respectability through cosmetic surgery in Finland. *Sociology Of Health & Illness*, 32(2), 258-271.
7   Ibid.
8   Ibid.

9   Covino, D. (2001). Outside-In: Body, Mind, and Self in the Advertisement of Aesthetic Surgery. *Journal Of Popular Culture*, 35(3), 91.

10   Suissa, A. (2008). Addiction to Cosmetic Surgery: Representations and Medicalization of the Body. *International Journal Of Mental Health & Addiction*, 6(4), 619-630.
11   Ibid.

12   Covino, D. (2001). Outside-In: Body, Mind, and Self in the Advertisement of Aesthetic Surgery. *Journal Of Popular Culture*, 35(3), 91.

Impact on Family

CHAPTER SEVEN

When I close my eyes and think about the different people in my life that I care about, I see a mental picture of them. I see my loved ones smiling at me. I see my brother smiling. I see my dad laughing. I see my sister and my mother talking. I see facial expressions and colors. I feel love warming my heart.

I know my family's laugh lines, hair color, skin tone, and body types. I can pick them out of a crowd just by noticing their stride and the way they hold their shoulders. There is something familiar in their look. Even as I look in the mirror, I see my parents and my brother and sister in my own reflection.

There is an intimacy that comes through knowing the "imperfections" that make us who we are. There is a comfort in familial traits. To value our body's imperfections is to value everything I just wrote about.

My father had a terrible accident in 2005. He fell 18 feet from a tree where he was cutting down limbs. He broke both hips, his sacrum, his arm, and his hand was almost totally disconnected from his body. He almost lost his hand, but thank God he didn't. The surgeon said the break was the worst he'd ever seen still connected to the body.

It was a traumatic experience, not only for my father, but for everyone in our family. I needed adjustment time after I saw my dad's crushed arm. It changed me. It grieved me seeing him go from running in the Army for 20 years, to being in so much pain everyday that he doesn't even want to take a walk.

Ten years later, I still struggle as I look at the large scar down his entire arm. I'm proud of him for moving forward, working through the pain, and gaining back his range of motion. But it took time to for me to adjust. It takes time to accept change.

A friend of mine told me about his friend who was in a terrible car accident. His face was scarred as a result. After multiple reconstructive surgeries, his friend is still suffering from the damage to his face. It discourages him when he sees how other people look at him with fear. At the same time, he's tired of surgery and isn't going to pursue it anymore.

Reconstructive and restorative surgeries can make a world of difference in the life of a physically traumatized person. Still, my mind goes to people who have embraced their body after trauma, and decided to use it to make a difference in the world.

I think of Dave Roever and other military heroes who move forward in the face of the physical trauma they survived. I think of Nick Vujicic and other people born some kind of difference that might be considered limiting. I think of Reshma Quereshi, a survivor of an acid attack—the mutilation of young women and girls by pouring acid on the face.

They are more than survivors. They are my heroes. They worked through the realities they face in the mirror everyday, accept their bodies, and even use their scars to challenge and change the world to be a better place.

What is different about their situation compared to ours? Where is their strength coming from? I'm in awe of these people that share their scars with the world.

Why is it that some of us are afraid to embrace brokenness? I am particularly talking to those of us who have *not* experienced trauma. Why are we so afraid to embrace what we consider physical flaws, both in ourselves and in others? I think it is because it brings us face to face with our vulnerabilities and weaknesses. It makes us uncomfortable because it reminds us we are human and that our lives can change in an instant. Cosmetic surgery may be a way that some of us run away from vulnerability. If we correct what we think is imperfect, we protect ourselves from potential rejection.

Would you love your child any more or any less if their teeth were straight or crooked? No. Do you love your husband less if his hair is gray or brown? No. Will you be more proud of your daughter if she is thinner? No. We aren't so superficial. Are we?

But what about making it better?

What if straightening your child's teeth will give her the confidence to hold her head up high and smile more? What if dying his hair will make your husband feel like taking you out on a romantic date more often? What if going on a diet would make your daughter feel better about her body?

These activities are socially acceptable, low-risk, and fairly inexpensive. They are tools we commonly use to "feel good" about ourselves. What would happen if we practiced "feeling good" about ourselves without using these simple outward changes that are easily within our reach?

Of course, we want the best for the people we love. We want them to feel their best, look their best, and be free to live their lives. We want to empower them, and we want them to take care of themselves. We want to be supportive in their pursuits. We may even want to financially help make their dreams come true.

Let's raise the stakes.

What if your parents' face-lift will bring back a sense of youthfulness, and help them feel more like they did when they self-actualized, when they were at their physical peak? Some people—both men and women—believe cosmetic surgery could benefit their careers, since people are working longer and competing with younger candidates. What if having surgery opened the door to allow your loved one to make more money? What if your teenage daughter would feel like a beautiful woman if she had breast implants? What if your young-adult child wanted a sex-change? What if your parents divorced and your mother transformed herself to look like a totally different woman?

Do we really want our loved ones to undergo cosmetic surgery to bring about feelings of self-worth? Do we want them to risk their lives to change their bodies? We must acknowledge the risks. The quote by Edelman[1] is worth repeating, "With our mania for surgery in this country, we seem to have blurred the distinction between toning up at the gym and having our thighs liposuctioned; between having a facial and a face lift . . . It is not the same thing, folks. Surgery can kill you."

Some older adults who undergo plastic surgery balk at the idea of their aging parents choosing cosmetic surgery.[2] We want it for ourselves, but why not for our family members? We would still love our family members, no matter what they did to their bodies, but would we experience a sense of grief if we knew we would never see the same image of the person we've grown to love, ever again?

If we eliminate the look of aging, we eliminate learning what it's like to embrace who we are as we age with grace. In trying to regain a sense of youthfulness, think of what we would lose in the process: the smile lines, the physical attributes we've come to know, the distinction that comes naturally with age.

Some would argue that we will lose our physical image regardless. There is a grieving process involved in watching our parents and children age. There's the possibility of trauma due to an accident or some other terrible situation that could steal a physical attribute away. We may have to face the initial shock of adjusting to their transformed bodies, scarred for life.

Your family members are worth considering as you make a choice about cosmetic surgery for yourself. We all are free to make our own choices, but there are always consequences to our choices. What we choose will not only alter us, but it will influence the people we love as well. How will your surgery change and challenge the people who love you?

What do your loved ones want for you? There is much more to altering physical attributes via surgery than there is to going to the spa for the day.

Just as there is an adjustment time to accepting the scars from trauma, there is a parallel adjustment time to accepting a surgical adjustment that is purely cosmetic. There is a sense of loss when we move from one bodily state to another, even if we perceive the change to be positive. With every change, there is a loss, and a time to grieve before moving forward into acceptance.

Cosmetic surgery can take a toll on our relationships. Relationships are fragile. Cosmetic choices are personal. These issues, though affecting our society as a whole, are family issues.

This entire relational chapter was the most difficult chapter for me to write. I put off writing it as long as I possibly could. Part of my hesitation in writing comes from the fact that I am not married, and do not have children. It's hard to write about how cosmetic surgery impacts marriage and family, considering I was a teenager when I had my surgery. Despite that, I have had the past 15 plus years to contemplate the many questions that have come to my mind concerning my own surgery and how it may potentially impact my future spouse and children. This chapter shares some of my own personal perspectives, but I also relied on much research.

Disclosing Cosmetic Surgery to Children

Whether or not to disclose cosmetic surgery to young children or teenagers is a controversial topic. Experts warn that a parent telling their child about their cosmetic surgery can influence the child's body image. The American Society for Aesthetic Plastic Surgery[3] reports that 7 to 12 percent of cosmetic surgery patients have some level of Body Dysmorphic Disorder (BDD), an obsessive psychological condition that can be passed down to children.

How will your child find out about your choice to have cosmetic surgery, and how will finding out affect them? Young children may be afraid if they see their parents' bruises, swelling, or scars. Surgeries may send the message that an inherited physical family feature is ugly and needs to be fixed in order to be acceptable.

On the other hand, children who do not know about their parent's surgeries may compare their features to that of their parents, and feel inadequate according to cultural standards of beauty when they don't measure up and their parents do.[4]

Not telling children could also potentially harm the parent-child relationship.[5] Elizabeth Berger, child psychologist and author of "Raising Kids with Character," said that while hiding the facts about a makeover may not be the same as lying, it can still violate trust within a relationship. Children are sensitive and can pick up on gut feelings, especially if the parent holds the attitude that they are hiding a dirty secret.[6]

A survey by the American Society for Aesthetic Plastic Surgery reported more than half of Americans approve of cosmetic surgery.[7] As the stigma associated with plastic surgery decreases, more and more children will have knowledge of their parents' surgeries. Our children's wellbeing is worth considering when making a decision about cosmetic surgery for ourselves, and disclosing our choices to them.

There is a danger of a parent's cosmetic surgery influencing children's view of body image and sexuality in negative ways. Dr.

Jim Taylor, a professional in child development and parenting, teaches that children are sponges for the early messages they receive. He warns that the bombardment of negative messages from popular culture may drown out healthier messages parents try to send. Taylor cites a recent study that found girls as young as six-years-old associated more with dolls who were dressed sexily if they spent a lot of time watching media, or if they had mothers who were overly invested in their own appearance.[8]

Taylor doesn't leave out a father's influence either. "Hey, don't forget us fathers either in whether or not young girls see themselves as sexual beings. If you don't think dads have an impact, you're being naive. Think about it. If you read men's magazines, ogle cheerleaders while watching football on TV, or get upset when your wife isn't all "dolled up," what messages are you sending to your daughters?"[9]

What about the impact of a parent's cosmetic surgery on sons? The same messages about self-worth and family physical features are passed on to sons as they are to daughters. Messages about sex are also passed on. What does it do to a son's view of sexuality when his mother has a breast enhancement surgery? What does it do to his mind when he has to adjust to seeing her body change all of a sudden. How does it impact the way he feels about women?

"When children are exposed to these messages enough, they can't help but internalize them and make them their own. And, sadly, these unhealthy messages shape the values, attitudes, and beliefs they come to hold about themselves and the world. It's not hard to see, then, how early exposure to sexuality can set [children] on an unhealthy life path," Dr. Taylor said.[10]

All is not lost. Parents can influence their children away from negative messages about sexuality and self-image regardless of if cosmetic surgery is a part of the family dynamic. The words of affirmation and quality time a father and mother give their children can go a long way in teaching them a healthy pattern of thought and approach to life, body image, and sexuality. Talking about cosmetic choices takes away the stigma, and allows a parent to shape the child's view of the surgery.

In my personal opinion, focusing on building a strong relationship built on honesty and trust is more important in a child's development than whether or not you choose to have a cosmetic procedure. There's a huge difference in openly talking about options, risks, and benefits, as opposed to hiding cosmetic surgery choices from a child, teenager, or adult child. God forbid, but what if you were to die during a cosmetic procedure? What good would hiding the surgery do then? How would your child approach processing your loss?

Knowing a parent trusts their child enough to be vulnerable about their own bodily complaints and decisions can build understanding and empathy. Hiding choices or pretending like they never occurred, despite the obvious, embodies a sense of shame and sends the message that the parent-child relationship lacks trust and intimacy.

Some people believe boundaries between parents and children should omit disclosing surgical decisions. They say it's "personal" and "private" and that children should not be exposed to adult decisions. Sadly, I believe these parents are missing the point. If they aren't talking to their children about real life, someone will. If you don't want your child knowing you personally, what quality of relationship are you aiming for?

When Your Kid Wants Cosmetic Surgery

I know a girl whose dad bought her breast implants for her sixteenth birthday. It's really not that uncommon. Would you give your child cosmetic surgery as a gift? I challenge you to ask yourself this question, particularly concerning your teens: does your kid want cosmetic surgery enough that if he or she had to work to pay for it, they would be willing to cover the cost?

I've asked myself if I would ever want my child to have cosmetic surgery. I have come to the conclusion that my answer is "No." Still, it is something I would have to weigh out with my future husband, depending on the situation. I continue to ask myself questions about the future. What will I tell my child when cosmetic surgery is even more popular than it is now?

What if your young child is experiencing bullying due to being teased over a physical feature, such as protruding ears? Otoplasty, ear surgery, is one of the only widely accepted surgeries for children, along with cleft lip and cleft palate surgery.[11] Of course, these fall more into the reconstructive or restorative types of surgeries versus cosmetic, but the questions we need to think about are the same.

One child was seven years old when she had surgery to pin back her ears. Her mother said the girl always received questions at school from other kids about her ears, but adults usually made the worst comments. The girl was very sensitive to all of the questions and taunts.[12]

Statistics from the American Society for Aesthetic Plastic Surgery show the number of children and teens who have cosmetic procedures has increased almost 30 percent over the past ten years, and experts believe the jump is in response to bullying.[13] There is controversy over the choice for cosmetic surgery in bullying cases as well. As one professional said, "We never want to hold the victim responsible for the bullying."[14]

To suggest cosmetic surgery to stop bullying is a passive response. Why should a perfectly healthy child feel he or she must conform via surgery in order to stop bullying? Surgery should be the last option, in my opinion. It is our job to protect our children, to fight their battles, to equip them to fight their own battles as they grow, and to provide a safe environment for them to have imperfections and still know they are fully loved as they are.

You know the circumstances your child is going through. I can't say what is right or wrong for your child and your child's situation. You know their maturity, what they can handle, and what is best for them. Prayerfully consider the options. Take your child to counseling. Find out what they really want and need. Don't opt for the quick-fix because that's the popular or "easy" solution. Do the hard work to make sure your child or teen is emotionally and relationally healthy before suggesting cosmetic surgery.

As I held a friend's little girl at a Bible study one night, I looked at her smooth skin, perfectly clear eyes, and ringlet hair. What would the little girl be like when she was a teenager? I thought. Would she know her worth? Would she overflow with life and beauty as she did as a toddler? Would she grow up knowing that God made her and loves her exactly how she is? Would she learn to function at her best and flow in the gifts God gave her? Or would she somehow become convinced she needed cosmetic surgery to be beautiful and capable?

I think of my future children, if the Lord blesses me with them. What can I do to teach them that they are naturally beautiful? I know I won't be able to control my children's thoughts or self-esteem. Ultimately, they will have to make their own choice in what they think and feel about themselves. No doubt, they will face their own inner struggles. But I will have an influence, and the way I live and think about myself will draw a pattern for them to follow.

I pray I can empower my children with healthy self-esteem by loving myself for who I am, and by fully enjoying and living life in pure worship to God. I am committing to my future children, that I will not verbalize my insecurities to them. I will never say, "I look fat." I will not talk about wrinkles, or age spots, or gray hair in a disparaging way.

I will age with grace. I will make it fun to be healthy and active. I will emphasize going, doing and being, not wishing, hoping and dreaming. I will validate what they care about, and hold them when they are afraid. I will teach them that they are beautiful by the way I live my life.

Cosmetic Surgery and Marriage

I have talked to a few women who have told me that having a breast enhancement was the best thing they have done for their marriage. They have no regrets and would make the choice again in a heartbeat. Some of these women said they feel more like "women" after breast enhancement, and their sexual confidence increased.

Other women have said their husband became jealous of their bodies after their surgeries. Some men accuse their wives of having an enhancement to gain the attention of other men. Still, other women say cosmetic procedures were a source of argument between them and their husbands, and caused problems in the relationship because their husbands didn't want them to have cosmetic surgery.

Dr. Richard Carlino, a plastic surgeon in North Carolina, precautions married women to take their husbands into consideration during the decision making process about cosmetic surgery. He gave the following statement in an article titled, *Will Plastic Surgery Save Your Marriage?*

> Everyone contemplating elective cosmetic surgery needs to do their homework. They should have all of their ducks in a row and not be borrowing from Peter to pay

Paul, should be at the right place in life — emotionally, financially, physically — and should not adhere to the philosophy that it is easier to ask forgiveness than permission. Have your spouse involved in the process. Women should be sure they are doing any [procedure] for themselves.... There is, however, a side to [having a spouse as a motive for cosmetic surgery]. A woman may have all of the right motives including doing it for herself and her husband. In a healthy relationship, both individuals should have a stake in the process.[15]

Another plastic surgeon, Dr. Rod Rohrich, will not perform cosmetic surgery on patients undergoing major life changes such as grieving a death or divorce. "I want to do it if the patient is doing it for themselves—not for their new boyfriend, or to save their marriage. I can't make a 5'1 woman into a D cup. Maybe that's what some want – and they can always get what they want somewhere else. But I turn them away."[16]

Some researchers say that from a survival of the fittest perspective, transforming the body with cosmetic surgery may be useful in acquiring important benefits, such as finding the ideal marriage partner.[17] Some women feel the need to use cosmetic surgery to keep their marriage partner. Knowing that breaks my heart for marriages in our generation.

I've noticed many older women who have undergone cosmetic surgery procedures. It's most obvious to me when I see these women walking around with their husbands. Typically, the man is balding, wrinkled, has a potbelly, and looks his age. The woman's face is taunt and wrinkle-free. Her facial expressions are limited. Her hair is blonde, her lips are red. She's had at least one face-lift, possibly an eye-lid surgery, breast implants that had to be replaced twice, and Botox every three months. The example may sound extreme, but if you look around, you'll probably see a similar couple.

I have to wonder why in many cases it is the female who chooses cosmetic surgery, while the male does not. I wonder if her husband's preferences had anything to do with her choices. Maybe it wasn't anything he said, but what he didn't say. Throughout the years, did he continue to tell his wife how beautiful she was to him? Did he make fun of other women's bodies, causing her to wonder what he thought about her body? I wonder how much their relationship impacted her choice to alter her body.

Abuse and Identity Crisis

There's an area of relational consideration I haven't written about yet, so I want to briefly bring it to your attention. I've written about female tendencies to use cosmetic surgery to find a mate. I've hinted at the idea that male pornography addictions influence female cosmetic choices. But I haven't mentioned sexual abuse.

We usually think of sexual abuse as the unwanted, or inappropriate touching or penetrating of a person's genital area. But that is not the only definition. Body shaming, sexual humor, sexual misinformation, and exposure to pornography are all considered sexual abuse.[18] There are even more issues, too extensive for the scope of this book—such as emotional incest, mind rape, humiliation, mental abuse, and all kinds of deviant and evil acts—that might influence a person's choice to have cosmetic surgery.

Sexuality is very much a part of our cosmetic choices. Recently, cosmetic surgery trends have shifted to altering genitals to produce a particular look. This type of cosmetic surgery is not the same as a sex-change resulting from a gender identity crisis. Women are having procedures called labiaplasty, or labioplasty, on their inner and outer labias. Males are undergoing penile enlargement implants.

We already know that female breast enhancement is the number one cosmetic surgery in the U.S. With the new trends in cosmetics on genitals, there is no doubt in my mind that all of these surgeries are connected to sexual brokenness. I have to wonder if pornography and sexual abuse has any influence in these situations. What I'm talking about is going on with heterosexual, "traditional marriage" types of people—yes, even in the Christian community.

I have barely mentioned the sexual and gender identity crisis in our country. To me, the stories of transgenders and their sex-changes are no different than the stories of heterosexuals who pursue cosmetic surgery. Many of our cosmetic surgery choices come down to one common denominator: brokenness at the core of who we are.

I have to continually emphasize that changing our bodies, no matter what part of the body we change, will not change who we are inside. Cosmetic surgery will not transform a person into a new soul. Cosmetic surgery must not be used as an answer for a personal identity crisis, relational crisis, or any other crisis. If anything, cosmetic surgery will compound the issues that a person in crisis is struggling to sort out. When we take our lives into our own hands, instead of placing our lives into the hands of our Creator, we end up sinking further and further away from God's plan.

Psalm 139:14

I praise you because I am fearfully and wonderfully made. Marvelous are Your works, and that my soul knows very well.

Questions for Reflection

- Have you talked to your child about cosmetic surgery?
- Is your child experiencing bullying? If yes, what have you done to confront and stop the bully, or help your child deal with the bully?
- Will you talk to your child about your cosmetic experiences and choices?
- What would you tell your daughter if she asked for a breast augmentation for her 16th birthday? Would it make a difference if the augmentation were a reduction versus an enhancement?
- How could cosmetic surgery benefit or harm your child's quality of life?
- What do you think the impact of a mother's breast enhancement is on a son or daughter's ideas about sex, pornography, and their own bodies, or future partner's bodies?
- If you are married, what is your spouse's opinion concerning cosmetic surgery? Have you talked to your spouse about your thoughts on cosmetic surgery?
- Are you considering cosmetic surgery for sexual reasons?
- Have you experienced any kind of sexual abuse, body shaming, name-calling, or sexual misinformation that is influencing your choice toward cosmetic surgery?
- Are you experiencing a crisis of any kind?

Endnotes

1   Edelman, H. S. (1994). Why is Dolly Crying? An Analysis of Silicone Breast Implants in America as an Example of Medicalization. *Journal Of Popular Culture, 28*(3), 19-32.

2   Kinnunen, T. (2010). 'A second youth': Pursuing happiness and respectability through cosmetic surgery in Finland. *Sociology Of Health & Illness, 32*(2), 258-271.

3   Surgery.org

4   Kubota, Taylor (2011). Parenting while plastic: A debate about how parents should disclose cosmetic surgery to their children. Scienceline.org. Accessed June 4, 2014. http://scienceline.org/2011/12/parenting-while-plastic
5   Ibid
6   Ibid
7   Ibid

8   Taylor, Jim (2012). The Disturbing Sexualization of Really Young Girls. Huffington Post. Accessed September 23, 2015 from www.huffingtonpost.com/dr-jim-taylor/the-disturbing-sexualization_b_1948451.html.
9   Ibid
10   Ibid

11   Carollo, K. (2011). When is Cosmetic Surgery the Answer to Bullying? ABC News. Accessed September 23, 2015 from abcnews.go.com/Health/cosmetic-surgery-answer-bullying/story?id=13255540.
12   Ibid
13   Ibid
14   Ibid

15   Beckman, J. (2011). Will plastic surgery save your marriage? *SheKnows*. Accessed September 23, 2015 from www.sheknows.com/love-and-sex/articles/841083/could-plastic-surgery-save-your-marriage.

16   Davis, J. (2008). How will breast implants change your life? WebMD. Accessed September 23, 2015 from www.webmd.com/beauty/breast-implants/how-will-breast-implants-change-your-life?

17 Suissa, A. (2008). Addiction to Cosmetic Surgery: Representations and Medicalization of the Body. *International Journal Of Mental Health & Addiction*, 6(4), 619-630.

18 Ferree, Marnie. (2013). *No Stones: Women Redeemed from Sexual Addiction*. InterVarsity Press. Downers Grove, IL.

Privacy, Secrecy, and the Church

CHAPTER EIGHT

I know I am not the only person who felt that cosmetic surgery was a shameful secret I needed to hide from members of my church. It's a very common perception. I once heard someone say there is a vast difference between privacy and secrecy. Keeping an issue private because it is personal is totally different than keeping a secret because you are afraid of the consequences, are avoiding intimacy, or are concerned you'll be judged.

My parents encouraged me to keep the matter of my surgery private because it was a personal issue. They felt it wasn't anyone else's business what I chose to do. I agree with them, and I am glad I didn't talk about my surgery around the time that it happened. I also think my parents did a good job of protecting me, and the family, from judgment.

At the time, their advice was correct. I was young and I needed to heal and psychologically process my facial changes before I was ready to publicly talk about it. As an adult, I understand the risk of talking about my past. I have stronger boundaries now, and I believe I am following God's plan for my life by sharing my story. I don't think I went through all of that physical and emotional pain for no reason. I believe my experience is for a greater purpose in God's kingdom. I want to use my story to give glory to God.

After my surgery, later that year, I was torn over my need to talk out my emotions to experience inner healing, and my desire to honor my parents' wishes and stay silent. I needed affirmation that I was "OK," so I did talk about my surgery with a couple of safe people—a teacher and a friend near my age. Thankfully, they listened to me without judgment. In fact, they didn't see what the big deal was to me, or why I even wanted to talk about it. They both expressed a desire to have cosmetic surgery on themselves.

I now understand my desire to talk about what I'd been through came from a place within me that needed emotional and relational healing. It wasn't about the surgery as much as it was my needing to feel connected, and know I wasn't alone. Back then there weren't a lot of "recovery" types of programs available that I was aware of, but something inside of me still knew that the way to heal was to talk about what I'd been through.

One of the motivational factors in my writing this book is my hope to launch respectful discussions on the topic and experience of cosmetic surgery. I hope this book will provide a launch pad for group discussion, and open the door for examining the many complex facets of our humanity as it relates to cosmetic surgery.

Secrecy at Church

Of all the places people are not willing to talk about plastic surgery, I think church is the number one. Christians undergo cosmetic surgery, but many of them are not talking about it. Some are even hiding it, or pretending it never happened. I understand

and respect individual unwillingness to talk about personal choices in a church setting. It's important to maintain boundaries and a sense of personal safety when discussing private matters. But if there is no teaching or talking about the subject, where can an individual go to learn or process questions they may have? Surely, among the millions of us that have had surgery, at least several thousand may want to attend a support group of some kind.

Considering the high number of surgeries taking place every year, I believe leaders should be aware of and willing to address the underlying spiritual and emotional issues potentially associated with cosmetic surgery. There are too many people spiritually bound to shame, inadequacy, and the quest for perfection. What if the church provided a place where people could find unconditional positive regard—love—and a safe environment to process their lives and heal from hurts. Isn't that what Jesus was about?

Many churches are currently participating in Celebrate Recovery types of programs, and tapping into the importance of confidentiality, raw honesty, and accountability. Other places of worship view the role of the church as strictly to provide theological teaching, prayer, and spiritual support. Churches that do not provide social or emotional care often refer their people to counselors to discuss personal issues. And then there are other churches that believe in dictating nearly every facet of members' lives, relegating them to conform to rules, and not caring much about the state of their heart.

Regardless of the type of church you belong to, I think it's important to have boundaries in place. Boundaries protect your privacy from unsafe people. Boundaries give you room to make an informed decision on whether or not to have cosmetic surgery without input from people who may want to influence you one way or the other.

There is a balance between privacy and secrecy. We have to know who is safe to talk to, and who is not—even in the church. There are some great and trusted resources on that topic, including the book *Safe People: How to Find Relationships That Are Good for You and Avoid Those that Aren't*, by two of my favorite authors, Dr. Henry Cloud and Dr. John Townsend.

Churchy Perceptions

Let me start with defining what I mean by church. I'm talking about the place you go every Sunday, the building filled with people, which has its own culture, norms, expectations, and unique group dynamics. I'm not talking about the Biblical sense of the church—meaning the bride of Christ, the true spiritual sons and daughters of God who have an actual relationship with our Creator. I'm talking about a social group of people in which the members influence each other.

Here are some questions to get you thinking about what your church is like. Do the people in your church have something positive to offer? What is it? Do the people in your church act like they have it all together, or are they open about their struggles? Are the people in your church sincerely following Christ and the Bible? Does your church have a formal stance on cosmetic surgery?

Within every denomination is a multiplicity of church dynamics. Each church congregation has a unique personality. Within every denomination we can find progressive and traditional churches, as well as churches in transition on the spectrum between conservative and liberal.

A pastor once gave the best definition I've ever heard of the difference between a "conservative" and a "liberal" church. He said, "If the other person thinks you are stricter than they are, they will label you as conservative. If they think you do less than they do for God, then they will label you as liberal." I've found his statement to be true.

After talking with my Hindu and Muslim friends, I feel safe in saying these same dynamics can be found in every religion. In a very human way, we all share the same experience of dealing with a variety of personalities, preferences, beliefs, and standards within our particular religious and cultural backgrounds. The social experience we all encounter is what sociologists and psychologists call basic group dynamics and subculture norms.

Social influence is important, and most everywhere we go there is pressure to change in order to be accepted. We can find peer pressure at school, church, work, and with family. Having an understanding of how a system operates, whether that system is an educational or religious system, social system, or a family system, is crucial to navigating and excelling within that system. When rules are clearly defined, it is easier to assimilate into a system. At the same time, clearly defined expectations put enormous pressure on people to conform or face rejection.

I believe it is important that a system define its rules and standards. Without making it clear, there is chaos and confusion. When a group is up front about what they stand for, they are doing everyone a favor and saying, "This is who we are." It is easier for outsiders to choose whether or not they want to be a part of the group. It's also easier for outsiders to feel discouraged in their search for a church when they feel they can't live up to particular ways.

It's no secret that many churches, especially traditional or more conservative churches, would consider cosmetic surgery morally questionable. Yet, even in the strictest of churches, people are undergoing cosmetic surgery—often keeping it a secret. It's happening, and it will continue to happen. Millions of people in the U.S. had cosmetic surgery last year. Surely there were quite a few conservative Christians among those patients. I know at least seven of them personally.

So when I ask the question, "How does the church influence decisions toward or against cosmetic surgery?" I am talking about **your** church. The church you attend, or have loose ties with, or the one you call your spiritual home. Mostly, I'm asking about the people you allow to influence your life.

Making Peace with God and Church

I grew up in what most people would consider a conservative home. When I was a child we didn't have a TV and we stayed away from what we called ungodly and worldly influences. I was raised to act and dress in a traditional way.

The churches my family attended emphasized modesty and being set apart from the world in the way we behaved, including the way we dressed. We were taught that living for God started on the inside, but eventually reflected on the outside. It was a big focus. The church emphasized purity and glorifying God with cleanliness and respectable living, which of course should reflect on the outside.

I've mentioned before that I didn't cut my hair growing up. In fact, the first time I trimmed it, I was 28-years-old. I had cosmetic surgery when I was 16. From age 16 to 28, I struggled spiritually to understand why it was okay to cut my face, but not my hair. I talked to a church lady about my feelings. Her only reply was, "We've done a great injustice to our children."

I made peace with God about my face and my hair. When I cut my hair I realized how *not* a big deal it was despite what many church people said. It was nothing like cutting my face. My hair grew out, and I trimmed it again. I felt no remorse or distance from God. It may seem like a small thing to you, but for me it was a milestone. I grew up being taught that God honored my prayers because I had never cut my hair, and that He saw my commitment, dedication, and submission by my honoring Him and church leaders through femininity and submission to authority—since He created me to be a female. I grew up believing that not cutting my hair was a part of honoring God as a woman.

After I cut my hair, I knew God loved me for me—not for my uncut hair. Yes, He saw my sincerity, my commitment, and my dedication, but that was a matter of heart, not of hair.

Not cutting my hair for such a long time taught me a lot. It taught me commitment, self-denial, and respect for other people's preferences. I can remember all the times I wanted to cut my hair, but pushed through my desires and stayed committed to the vow I had made as a child. That type of discipline goes a long way, and translates to other areas of life. Not cutting my hair taught me how to stay committed and faithful through difficult times, even when I don't feel like it.

I still have long hair. I love my hair, and I love being feminine. I am who I am, and I choose to look the way I look because this is me—not because I am trying to please anyone. I'm not dressing to please other people anymore. I'm just being me, and living life the way I feel at peace with God.

The ironic thing is, a lot of people who "do less" than me sometimes still treat me as if I was so different from them. At the same time, those that "do more" than I do often treat me as if I'm a liberal. None of that matters anymore, though. I'm just me. I will fit-in with kind and good people no matter how they dress or what they believe.

Finding a Church

Growing up, I tried so hard to be a good person, to follow every rule and to please the people I thought of as spiritual authority in my life. Despite my best efforts, there were times I still met judgment and rejection. My heart breaks for people who strive for love and acceptance within the church and are met instead with judgment and social rejection. I know what it feels like to be socially outcast in a church of my own denomination.

Thankfully, because I have moved around a lot, I've seen a lot of amazing, kind, and true Christians within my denomination, along with the bad ones. I've been able to move forward and find people and places where I do belong. But sometimes it takes going through a difficult situation in order to find an amazing one.

I was a young adult on my own looking for a church to attend in the new town I just moved to. It was my first Sunday to visit a particular church, but I knew several people who attend there. I didn't know the pastor or his wife personally, so I was shocked when the pastor's wife approached me and told me that makeup wasn't allowed in their church. I was wearing natural-looking face powder. She then informed me that I had a "spirit of Jezebel." I told her that was not the case, and that I disagreed with her. She didn't seem pleased with me after that, but I knew the truth about myself and wouldn't let her bully me into conforming.

I knew that pastor's wife didn't know me. She didn't know the loneliness and pain I'd suffered. She didn't know I had changed my face with cosmetic surgery. She judged me based on the outside, on a bit of powder. She had no idea of how far God had brought me in life, or what I had been through.

There were several other comments and experiences that happened at that church that were not right. At first, I tried to overlook the issues, hoping I was misreading these people, and that it was all in my imagination. I thought once I got to know the people better, my perception would change.

I stayed for as long as I could—a few months. That church, even though they believed the same theology I believed, was emotionally and spiritually abusive and an unsafe place. The church was doing more harm than good in my life, so I left.

I wonder how a church can consider itself the body of Christ if the culture is one of complete conformity, or total rejection? I've heard church leaders push for "holiness and submission," all the while causing damage, and breaking the hearts of sincere people who leave feeling ostracized and condemned.

There is no authentic ministry, love, or growth in veiling imperfections and struggles behind conformity in the name of obedience to authority. Quite the opposite, true Christians don't hide behind a mask of perfection, but admit their desperate need for a Savior.

For sure, no church is perfect, but the particular church I mentioned triggered pain in my heart. It wasn't a good fit for me. I knew it was not a safe place for me, and that I needed to leave. I needed to find a place where I would belong. I had to find a place where the imperfections didn't hurt me, a place where I could find healing and hope.

Around the time I left that church, I started praying about why the people there acted the way they did. I could tell that they were sincerely doing their best to live for God despite the negative behavior. They seemed to experience a demonstration of God's miraculous power in their worship services. Individuals found salvation at that church. Yet the emotional, social, and spiritual problems were so evident to me that it made me sick to my stomach and I had to leave.

God answered my prayer and led me to a scripture that helped me see the situation in a different light. The verse was Hebrews 4:12.

Hebrews 4:12 KJV
For the word of God is quick, and powerful,
and sharper than any two-edged sword,
piercing even to the dividing asunder
of soul and spirit, and of the joints and marrow,
and is a discerner of the thoughts and intents of the heart.

As I meditated on that verse, a word of wisdom whispered truth to my heart. **The people experienced God's presence because He loves them, but they have major soul problems they aren't dealing with.**

God spoke to my heart and helped me to understand a person can be spiritually saved by trusting in Christ, but still be emotionally and socially sick. It's the same as a person who has a physical cancer. Just because they are spiritually saved through faith, doesn't mean they won't get sick and die. A person can have faith in God and have other issues that need serious work. None of us are perfect. "For the wages of sin is death; but the gift of God is eternal life through Jesus Christ our Lord" (Romans 6:23 KJV).

After I left the hurt-church, I went to a healing-church. Just a few minutes away, I found a church I could call "home." The very next church I visited was one of the most well-rounded, loving places I've ever attended. The church was balanced in its ministry, totally out of debt, racially diverse, and affirming of both men and women in ministry.

I had an amazing experience at the second church. I played the piano, helped out with the young people, and was free to worship God without feeling judged. I knew I was appreciated, and I knew I made a difference. I had a pastor and pastor's wife whom I loved dearly, and they loved me.

God had a place for me where I would fit in, and I didn't have to change one thing about myself. I just had to be willing to step out after being hurt and find a place I fit. I learned not to give up on church altogether just because I experienced one that was abusive.

Finding Healing in God

I've heard the saying many times that "hurt people hurt people." I'm sure the people that hurt me at church are hurting inside. After experiencing the church abuse, I knew I needed to protect and care for myself, or I would end up hurting other people out of bitterness and anger because "hurt people hurt people."

A few years ago I heard an amazing second part of that quote. It said, "healed people heal people." Wow. I want to be a healed person that extends and hands of healing to the world around me. Jesus healed people. We are his hands and feet. When we embody

His healing power, we can bring health and healing to people around us.

Luke 2:52 (KJV) reads, "And Jesus increased in wisdom and stature, and in favor with God and man." My prayer is to seek Biblical wisdom to grow spiritually (God's favor), and to seek emotional and social health (favor with man). I want to be a light that points back God's grace and healing power.

Over time, I learned that the approval, or lack of approval, from church leaders and members could not complete me. Being good and following all of the rules wasn't enough to bring a sense of love into my life. As I learned these lessons, I realized my perception of how some church members acted toward me had seeped into my beliefs about God's love.

One day, as I was praying alone in my house, I begged God, "Please help me to be a better person so I will please You. Please, God I want you to love me."

As I said the words aloud, I realized that though I knew in my mind that God loved me, in my heart I didn't believe it.

I knew the scriptures. I knew God loved me. I felt ashamed that I begged God to love me. It was as if I dishonored Him by believing He didn't love me.

I don't know when it happened, but the love of God that I felt so strongly as a child seemed so far away. It was my heart and my love that was cold, and perhaps the love of the people around me that was cold—but not God's love. I just had to find it again.

That's when God's grace came and flooded my soul. The Holy Spirit gently reminded me of 1 John 3:20 and Matthew 24:10-14.

1 John 3:20 KJV
*Even when your heart condemns you,
God is greater than your heart . . .*

Matthew 24:10-14 KJV
And then shall many be offended, and shall betray one another, and shall hate one another. And many false prophets shall rise, and shall deceive many. And because iniquity shall abound, the love of many shall wax cold. But he that shall endure unto the end, the same shall be saved.

I began to realize that no matter how well I performed, no matter how good a person I was, no matter how holy or righteous, or abiding by the Bible I might be—my physical body would never walk on streets of gold. Heaven isn't like earth; my body would not survive there. In Heaven, I'll have a new body that God makes me—one that will be perfect. There's nothing I can do to create a perfect body, or soul, on earth—I'm totally dependent on God.

No matter how filled with the Holy Spirit I am, no matter how long I pray and commune in the depths of God's love, I still need His grace to go to Heaven. My righteousness is comparable to a filthy rag (Isaiah 64:6). I'm totally dependent on God's goodness, on His mercy, and on His power. And that is the best place I can be.

Relief flooded my soul and the power of the love of God brought me to tears. I could stop trying to be good and start focusing on the love of my Savior! I could live free from the anxiety of not being perfect! God loved me and He allowed me to feel His love in my soul.

Romans 8:38-39 KJV
I am persuaded, that neither death, nor life, nor angels, nor principalities, nor powers, nor things present, nor things to come, nor height, nor depth, nor any other creature, shall be able to separate us from the love of God, which is in Christ Jesus our Lord.

I think many of us have been hurt by church. We've been hurt by imperfect people who are hurt themselves. There is only one way for us to change the situation, and stop the cycle of abuse from continuing. We must finding healing in God, and start facilitating that healing for other people.

The wonderful part about imperfections is that it provides a time and place for a miracle to happen. Without a need, there will never be a reason for God to meet the need.

There is a need for people who are healed and full of love to start helping people who are hurting. It's time we start accepting each other, being the safe place, being the confidant someone else can turn to, and bearing each other's burdens.

Whether you chose cosmetic surgery or not, if you are an authentic and safe person, your life and choices can help create safety, and emotional and spiritual health for someone else. There are hurting hearts all around us that need authenticity and love in their imperfections. Let's move forward in being the real church, and making sure shame and secrecy have no place among us.

Questions for Reflection

- Are you fighting a spirit of worthlessness or shame concerning cosmetic surgery?
- Are you a part of a church where you feel loved and accepted? God loves you, but does your church love you?
- What is your local church's beliefs about plastic surgery?
- Does your church provide the authentic support you need to heal from any heart wounds you may have?
- I've heard my dad say several times, "Some people have 'daddy issues' with God; other people have 'mommy issues' with the church." Some people love God, but stay away from church because they've been hurt by church people. Sometimes going to church triggers pain. If you have church hurts, will you join me in starting the process of forgiving the church?
- If you have experienced spiritual and emotional abuse from people at church, do you have a place you can go to connect with safe people who can help you heal? It doesn't have to be a church or Christians who help you heal. With healthy boundaries, you can maintain your spiritual beliefs and still find healing through connection with healthy people who believe differently than you do. Who are the safe and emotionally healthy people in your life?

Shamefaced

CHAPTER NINE

I personally know ten other people who have had some type of cosmetic surgery. Only one of those other people speaks publicly about her surgeries. I heard her speak at a Christian women's conference about her addiction to cosmetic surgery, which occurred prior to her conversion. I spoke to her after the service, thanked her for her authentic honesty, and I told her about my surgery.

Many people feel ashamed about cosmetic surgery, and go to great lengths to hide the fact they did it. I've met Christian women who would rather die than openly admit they had a cosmetic procedure. One woman I met compared breast implants to tattoos of the '60s. She said it was a fad that everyone was doing, but then later you think, "Now, why did I do that?"

Outside of church, I've seen a few TV shows that discussed the issue, but the programs were mostly designed to promote plastic surgery. I've also noticed a great sense of shame connected to cosmetic surgery outside of the church. We want other people to think we are beautiful, but we don't want them to know we had surgery to make us more beautiful. None of us want to be seen as insecure or obsessed with our looks. We attach to shame without ever giving anyone else a chance to shame us. We shame ourselves.

When I had cosmetic surgery, I didn't want to shame my family. I also didn't want to shame God. I was afraid that talking about my surgery would sabotage my ministry before it had a chance to begin. It might even hurt my dad's ministry if people knew what his daughter had done.

What is shame? Merriam-Webster defines shame as "a feeling of guilt, regret, or sadness because of wrongdoing. The ability to feel guilt, regret, or embarrassment. Dishonor or disgrace." Shame is a feeling. It's an emotion. It's not a sin to feel shame, though true shame is often a result of sin in our lives. Sometimes we feel shame because of fear of judgment or rejection.

We all make choices in life that we regret and feel shame about. If you haven't, I have to wonder if you've really lived. Feeling shame is a human experience. Staying in shame, or moving forward away from it, is a choice.

I spent years in shame, afraid of judgment, and beating myself up for being insecure. I even felt ashamed for being human and having the need and desire to feel beautiful and loved. If I didn't look "just right" I felt ashamed. Throughout my teenage years, I would not go out of the house without make-up on, even though I've always been light on the make-up.

Once I grew out of my "home-schooled prairie-girl" look, as a teenager and young adult I had a lot of fun dressing up. Fashion became a hobby for me. I loved to go shopping and use my creativity to put together fun outfits. I had to have the high-heeled shoes, matching purse, pretty outfit, and great hair. I spent hours washing, drying, curling, and styling my hair in order to obtain "the look" I wanted. I felt proud walking into church knowing I achieved every requirement both for modesty and fashion. (Oh, the irony of feeling "proud" walking into church.) I received many compliments, and I took them to heart. If I didn't get a compliment, I must not have it together enough, I thought.

Once my family went on a trip to attend a large church conference. I remember being at the hotel getting ready to leave. As I worked on my hair, my dad made a comment I'll never forget. "You spend more time fixing your hair than you do praying," he said. His words cut straight to my heart. What he said was true. My life revolved around the way I looked, and trying to make myself more beautiful. I consciously knew I didn't want to live my life focused on my looks, but it was not easy to actually change. Despite learning to project confidence, insecurity consumed me.

Thankfully, God had a purpose in my insecurity, cosmetic surgery, and all of the healing that has subsequently come. I'm glad I learned my lessons, or I might still be stuck in the bathroom working on my hair! It motivates me to know God has a purpose and a plan for my life, and can use me no matter what.

The Shamefaced Woman

The churches I grew up in emphasized "shamefacedness" as a positive quality for a woman to have. Shamefacedness is an old word used in the King James translation of 1 Timothy 2:9. It is used as a part of the description of what a Christian woman should be like. But there is a problem when we tell women to be "shamefaced" because many of our generation hear only the word "shame." Our current understanding of the word "shame" is different from the original Greek word that was translated to "shamefacedness."

When we use the word "shamefaced" today it sounds as if we are saying women should be ashamed of their face, or should walk around with their head held low in shame. That is not what the Bible word for shamefaced means at all. If we are going to align ourselves with the Word of God, we have to take the time to understand the cultural context and original definition of Bible words.

Before I break down the original meaning of "shamefaced," I want to share a few different translations, or versions, of 1 Timothy 2:8-10.

King James Version: *I will therefore that men pray every where, lifting up holy hands, without wrath and doubting. In like manner also, that women adorn themselves in modest apparel, with* **shamefacedness** *and sobriety; not with broided hair, or gold, or pearls, or costly array; But (which becometh women professing godliness) with good works.*

The Message: *Since prayer is at the bottom of all this, what I want mostly is for men to pray—not shaking angry fists at enemies but raising holy hands to God. And I want women to get in there with the men* **in humility** *before God, not primping before a mirror or chasing the latest fashions but doing something beautiful for God and becoming beautiful doing it.*

The Living Bible: *So I want men everywhere to pray with holy hands lifted up to God, free from sin and anger and resentment. And the women should be the same way, quiet and sensible in manner and clothing. Christian women should be noticed for being **kind and good**, not for the way they fix their hair or because of their jewels or fancy clothes.*

When I researched the original meaning of "shamefaced," this is what I found. The Greek word used is *aidōs,* and means a sense of shame or honor, modesty, bashfulness, reverence, regard for others, and respect.[1]

The word *aidōs* is only found twice in the New Testament. In Hebrews 12:28, *aidōs* is translated to the English word "reverence." In light of the true meaning of the word shamefaced, here is how I apply 1 Timothy 2:9 to my own identity.

As a Christian woman, I want to be known for my reverence toward God and respect for other people, not for what I look like, how I dress, or for how beautiful I am.

The scripture doesn't mean I can not be beautiful, or that I can not wear nice clothing, or braid my hair, or wear jewelry. It means that my relationship with God will outshine the way I look. It means my life will not be wrapped up in if I'm having a good hair day, or bad one. My life won't be about if I'm happy with my body or not. My outward appearance won't influence my commitment to God, or how I treat other people. I want to be more concerned with my prayer life than looking good.

The Purpose of Shame

I think God allows us to feel shame for a reason. Just like pain has a purpose, shame has a purpose. Pain captures our attention and lets us know there is something wrong that needs tended to. Shame is the same way. It's a feeling that let's us know something is wrong, or something needs our attention. The emotion "shame" can't be denied. It is powerful, and we feel it to the core. Jesus understands our feelings of shame because He experienced them.

Hebrews 4:15 KJV

For we have not an high priest which cannot be touched with the feeling of our infirmities; but was in all points tempted like as we are, yet without sin.

Jesus died for our sin and He carried our shame with Him to the cross. In my lifetime of active church involvement, I thought I had heard a verse about Jesus' death on the cross being for our sin and shame. I thought I'd read it, but when I went to find it, there is no such verse. I think I was confused and thinking of Hebrews 12:2.

Hebrews 12:2 KJV

Looking unto Jesus the author and finisher of our faith; who for the joy that was set before him endured the cross, despising the shame, and is set down at the right hand of the throne of God.

Wow. Jesus felt the emotion of shame. He didn't die for our shame, but despised it as he endured it on the cross. If shame is an indicator of sin in our lives, and Jesus never sinned, then He had never felt shame prior to the cross. When He took our sin upon Himself, He experienced the feeling of shame for the first time, and He hated it! Shame is a terrible feeling to live with.

Jesus died for our sin, but it's our job to repent and accept forgiveness. If you are experiencing shame in relation to cosmetic surgery, perhaps due to a sin that fueled your decision, I pray you would allow God's power to transform your shame into shamefacedness—reverence for God and respect for people.

There is a beautiful place we can come to in experiencing the love and grace of God when we are honest about our feelings and regrets in life. I have never felt the love and grace of God as strongly as I do when I contemplate my regrets and realize that shame is gone—replaced by reverence and awe for God.

Romans 5:20 KJV

Where sin abounded, grace did much more abound.

If we are more concerned with the outside than we are with our hearts, that is truly something to be ashamed of. Let us not make idols of ourselves. Idolatry is sin.

Materialism can go to an extreme in more than one way. We can be consumed with wanting to look beautiful and be in style, or we can be consumed with wanting to look "holy" like a "good

Christian." Either way, if our main focus is on the outside and our looks, then we aren't focused on Christ.

I want to share my rendition of the story of the adulterous woman, found in John Chapter 8. It is a story about a sinful woman, who no doubt felt shame. It is the story of a woman who traded her shame for awe toward God. I've used my creativity to imagine why the story happened as it did.

The woman stood before Jesus in the place where she was condemned to die. I can imagine her screams as she was pulled out of bed and dragged through the streets. She had regrets. She knew she was guilty.

Jesus challenged the people who were ready to stone the woman. *"He who is without sin, cast the first stone!"*

One by one, the woman's accusers turned around and walked away.

I would think this woman would have fled to safety as soon as the people dropped their stones and left, but she didn't. There was only one accuser left. It was the woman herself.

Alone with Jesus, she stayed in the place of accusation, shame, condemnation, and punishment. She stayed because she accused herself. She stayed because she was guilty. She stayed in the place of torment because she believed she deserved to suffer and die.

Jesus did not leave the woman in the place of condemnation. He met her there.

He knelt in the dirt. Why such a humble position? Maybe He didn't want to intimidate or frighten her. Maybe He wanted her to see Him, but as long as she hung her head in shame, she wouldn't be able to see Him. He had to get low to the ground.

"Has no one condemned you?" He asked.

"No one, Lord," she answered.

"Neither do I condemn you. Go and from now on, sin no more."

Like the woman in the story, you may be in a place of shame over what you have done in life. Jesus is right there with you. He is there to deliver you from shame, just as He delivered me.

Remove yourself from the place of accusation. Remove yourself from the place of torment, and punishment, and death. Go, and live, and sin no more.

Let Psalm 119:133 be our prayer. *"Order my steps in thy word: and let not any iniquity have dominion over me."* Let no guilt, no shame, no feelings of unworthiness have dominion over us. If those feelings ever try to take over, help us to remember 1 John 3:20. *"When your heart condemns you, God is greater than your heart..."*

Questions for Reflection

- Do you feel a sense of shame and secrecy related to cosmetic surgery?
- If you feel shame connected to your cosmetic surgery, is it possible that shame is an indicator of a sin connected to your choice to alter your body?
- Is there any attitude or spirit attached to your choice that you need to repent of, and accept God's grace and forgiveness from?
- Do you feel the love and grace of God covering you?
- Are you ready to cultivate a deeper relationship with God that will allow His love and grace to free you from shame? He is with you. He loves you.

Endnote

1 BlueletterBible.org

Nothing New

CHAPTER TEN

Ecclesiastes 1:9 KJV
The thing that hath been, it is that which shall be; and that which is done is that which shall be done: and there is no new thing under the sun.

Throughout history and still today, some cultures use body-modification as a ritual or a rite of passage—a ticket to adulthood. For instance, some African tribes use facial scarring to easily identify who belongs to whom. Other cultures use body-alteration as a way to rise in social status, or make themselves more desirable as a marriage partner.

Many of the body-altering practices around the world and throughout history only happened with women. Do you remember seeing a picture of the Kayan Lahwi tribal women who placed coils around their necks to stretch their necks out long and tall? What about the stories of foot-binding that happened to young girls in China's history? Or the tiny waists of Victorian corset-wearing Western women? Sometimes these traditions led to death: broken necks with the removal of the coils, broken backs in child-birth after corsets wasted back muscles away, and the inability to walk due to broken, bound feet.

Sometimes body alteration isn't about social status, but about keeping women oppressed. I've heard stories of women in Asia and the Middle East who were punished with facial trauma for refusing an arranged marriage—some receiving acid thrown in their face. Then I've read of women who purposefully scar their own faces to protect themselves from kidnapping and forced marriages. Some women and girls are painfully circumcised, their bodies cut away at so they feel pain as they are raped by husbands who are sometimes twice or three times their age.

There are abuses in this world that are so atrocious our Western minds cannot even begin to imagine what life is like for these women. I view many of the body-altering practices around the world as barbaric and mutilating. I see these tragedies that happen to women overseas as acts of misogyny—hatred toward women.

I feel grateful as I sit writing a book about cosmetic surgery in a culture where I am free to write, free to speak, and free to stand up and say something meaningful. Of all the women throughout time and space, our generation of women in the Western world have the most freedom. We are free to seek education, own property, marry, or stay single. We are free to vote, run for office, and to spend our money the way we wish. We are free to change our bodies, and free to think about ourselves in whatever way we choose. We have more opportunity and more freedom than most women since the beginning of time.

But even in America, in our freedom, many women are financially oppressed by social systems, by bully-bosses on power trips, and by sexual harassment. To make it as a power-woman in the corporate world, many women throw away femininity, lockdown their emotions, and try to operate as men. On the other extreme in the corporate world, many women use sex to get a promotion or a raise.

Women who don't pursue a career are often financially dependent on men to the point they believe they cannot leave an abusive relationship. Low-income women lack education and support to change their circumstances. Single mothers make up the lowest income people-group in our country; many of their men are locked up in prison.

Women, from the ghettos to the gated communities, are often trapped by false-beliefs about their worth.

If Western culture prides itself on gender equality and women's empowerment, why are women the primary patients undergoing cosmetic surgery? Why are women's healthy bodies being cut and changed? Why are women spending weeks recovering from the trauma of surgery? Why is so much time, energy, effort, and money going into putting women's lives at risk to alter their bodies?

Some low-income women may not be able to afford expensive surgical procedures, but will spend the little money they have on a professional manicure every few weeks. In prison, men and women find a way to tattoo themselves, even though it is highly unsanitary.

I read about a low-income woman who wanted to change her bodies so much she risked illegal and unsafe back-ally surgeries. She allowed a "street surgeon" to inject fillers into her body to enhance her posterior. After two sessions, the woman rethought her decision and went to a doctor. She learned she was injected with bathroom caulk. She lived in pain for five years, and later developed a staph infection, which led to the amputation of her arms and legs.[2]

An article in *The New Yorker* claims that though the United States has the highest total number of cosmetic procedures, it is only number six when it comes to surgeries per capita. The article claims South Korea has one of the highest rates of plastic surgery per capita around the world, with Brazil at second place.[1]

A college student gave a quote for *The New Yorker* article about the general thoughts on cosmetic surgery in South Korea. "When you're nineteen, all the girls get plastic surgery, so if you don't do it, after a few years, your friends will all look better, but you will look like your unimproved you," she said. The article said it was common for men and women in their 20's and 30's to be out and about, even going to work with swollen faces and bandages from a recent procedure.

The Feminist Perspective

Feminist research critical of plastic surgery views the act as one that keeps women subordinate and classified as objects.[3] One woman, a 56-year old professor, regretted her choice to have a face-lift and eyelid surgery because it went against her values as an academic woman who believed her self-respect should not be based on her looks. Like that woman did, sometimes we make choices that clash with our true beliefs.

Cosmetic surgery can be an act of misogyny if a woman hates herself. There is a spiritual parallel between the cutting of our bodies and the damage hidden in our scarred souls. The enemy of our soul hates God's creation. Satan seeks to steal, kill, and destroy everything God creates from the inside out. We are under spiritual and emotional attack in our self-worth, body image, and confidence.

When it comes to cosmetic surgery, who really pays the price? Men may be paying for it financially, but everyone involved is sacrificing something. Cosmetic surgery is impacting everyone—the culture, the women, the children, and the family. There is a scar put on the soul with every cut that is made on the body. There is a story behind every surgery. Our circumstances are vastly different, but our hearts are so very much the same.

Pour Your Heart Out to God

Joel 2:13 NLT

Don't tear your clothing in your grief,
but tear your hearts instead. Return to the Lord
your God, for he is merciful and compassionate,
slow to get angry and filled with unfailing love . . .

Every body-altering act holds a deeper meaning. There is a reason behind every tattoo. Every mark and every cut tells the story of a life. Every cutter has a reason for slicing their wrists: a heartbreak, a pain, a desperation. Every person that pursues cosmetic surgery has a story. There is a reason why we alter our bodies.

In the Old Testament, when a person experienced a loss, in their grief they would rip their clothes, cut their hair, or shave their beard as an outward sign of inner heartbreak. They would often fast from eating food, and cover their head in ashes as a sign of their grief and humility.

In our culture today, for some of us, our pain is so deep we rip our bodies. We cut ourselves and throw away the parts we don't like. If you are basing your decision for cosmetic surgery on grief or emotional pain of any kind, I would like to suggest one thing before you continue: **Tear your heart (break open and pour your heart out to God) instead of tearing your body. Turn unto the Lord your God: for he is gracious and merciful, slow to anger, and of great kindness.**

The Bible compares our earthly bodies to a tent, a temporary dwelling place before moving to our permanent home. One day, we will put on heavenly bodies as if they were brand new sets of clothes. I know we all enjoy the feeling of finding a new outfit that we like. It's refreshing to have a facial, fix our hair, and clean up our nails, but all of these actions are temporary. None of them will last.

Even cosmetic surgery will not last. One day, no matter how hard we fight it, we will age, and our physical bodies will die. But when that day comes, those of us who are making our home with Jesus will have a new body.

That new body will never grow old, or need any kind of makeover. When we are in Heaven with the Lord, our earthly body will no longer be an issue. We will change our clothes from these worn out, patched up rags, and we will put on new life, and enter a heavenly body—one God Himself creates just for us.

2 Corinthians 5:1-5 NLT

For we know that when this earthly tent we live in is taken down, when we die and leave these bodies, we will have a home in heaven, an eternal body made for us by God himself and not by human hands. We grow weary in our present bodies, and we long for the day when we will put on our heavenly bodies like new clothing. For we will not be spirits without bodies, but we will put on new heavenly bodies. Our dying bodies make us groan and sigh, but it's not that we want to die and have no bodies at all. We want to slip into our new bodies so that these dying bodies will be swallowed up by everlasting life. God himself has prepared us for this, and as a guarantee he has given us his Holy Spirit.

Blood

Leviticus 17:11 ESV

For the life of the flesh is in the blood . . .

When I think about my own cosmetic surgery, I don't think about blood very much. I was not awake when the surgeon cut my body. I didn't see any blood, but blood was there. My blood, even just a little bit of it, was spilled out on that surgery table.

Blood is involved in many significant events in life. There is blood involved in childbirth. There is blood when the umbilical cord is cut. There is blood when we donate it to save a life. There is blood in an organ transplant. There is blood in a car-accident that claims a life. There is blood involved in significant life-changing events.

In the Bible when God made a covenant with His people, blood was involved. There was blood involved in circumcision, animal sacrifice, and ultimately on the cross at Calvary. In this section, I want to highlight the ancient world of "cutting covenants."

The Hebrew word for *"making"* as used in *"making a covenant"* is KRT, or "Karath." It means: "to cut off, to destroy or consume, to covenant or make agreement by cutting flesh and walking between the pieces."[4] Let me clarify, "the pieces" of flesh refer to the cut in-half pieces of animal flesh. It was a common practice in ancient times, not only in Israel but also in other nations and people groups, to make a covenant (a promise) by cutting an animal in half. As an animal lover, I do not like thinking about the reality of what happened to those poor creatures.

The covenant-makers would lay one half of the animal on one side of the road and the other half of the animal on the other side of road. The people would walk through the two halves of the animal to make a covenant. What they were essentially saying was, "If I break my end of the deal then let me be as this animal is—cut in half."[5]

Bruce William Jones, a retired professor from California State University's Religious Studies Department, wrote that ancient cutting rituals were used in making treaties, forming bonds, and as a part of blessings and curses. Cutting covenants could have been where the idiom "let's cut a deal" comes from.

The ancient Assyrian King Esarhaddon wrote a "cutting curse," which he read to his people as he cut open a baby lamb. He threatened to cut open any servant or soldier that deserted him or his son. The brutality set before the people brought a lot of fear. The ancient people tortured animals as a threat of what they would do to "rebels" who would not conform.

It's scary. It's not something I want to think about. I am so glad I wasn't born in those times. But that is how "cutting covenants" began.

God's Cutting Covenants

When Adam and Eve sinned, God cut an animal to clothe them. That animal's death was the first recorded death since the beginning of creation. Sin brought death into the world in more than one way.

Long before Israel was a nation, God formed a "cutting covenant" with Abraham, who was at that time called Abram. The story is found in Genesis 15. God tells Abram to bring Him a heifer, a goat, a ram, a turtledove and a pigeon. Abram "divides" (cuts in half) the larger animals and lays the pieces apart, next to each other.

Later that night, God spoke to Abram in a dream and told him that his descendants would endure four hundred years of slavery, after which He would bless them, and take them to the Promised

Land. To complete the covenant (promise), the Bible says "a smoking furnace and a burning lamp" passed between the pieces of the animals. Many theologians agree that the fire in this passage is a symbol of God, as it is in many other passages of scripture.[6] In this story God is essentially saying, "cut me in pieces if I fail to withhold my promises."

Circumcision

In Genesis 17, we see the first instance of the most well-known ritualistic cutting covenant in the Bible—circumcision. In the Old Testament, physical circumcision of males was the outward sign of being in covenant with God. Verse 13 says, "and my covenant shall be in your flesh for an everlasting covenant." As they made their covenant with God, Abraham and the men of his household cut their bodies. The cut in their flesh set God's people apart from pagans.

Cutting the Uncut

Along with the "cutting covenants," there were some instances where God's law required rituals specifically involving "cutting the uncut." Sacrificial animals were required to be whole and have no evidence of physical trauma. For example, Leviticus 22:24, "Ye shall not offer unto the Lord that which is bruised, or crushed, or broken, or cut; neither shall ye make any offering thereof in your land."

The Nazarite vow was another example. Volunteers who participated in the Nazarite vow took an oath to consecrate their bodies to God for a period of time, which could range from 30 days to a lifetime. Among several other requirements, the Nazarite was to keep his or her hair uncut. At the completion of the vow, the person cut their hair and presented it to God in a burnt offering.[7]

An Altar of Sacrifice

What happened back in the ancient times when there was a sacrifice? The people built an altar. It was a place where the flesh-cutting of animals occurred. It was a place where covenants were cut, and blood was spilled—sometimes resulting in death and sometimes not.

How many of us have ever been to an altar of sacrifice? I would say not many, if any of us. It's different today. God isn't looking for a bloody sacrifice—He took care of that at Calvary. God manifested Himself in human form to provide an atoning sacrifice for the sins of humanity (John 1 and 1 John 2). He gave His body to be broken (cut) for us, and His blood—His life—makes atonement for our sin (1 John 2:2).

We find eternal life in Christ's blood. We apply the blood of Jesus to our hearts when we kneel in repentance, looking to the cross of Christ as the atonement for our sin. We become a living sacrifice, holy, and acceptable for spiritual worship as we kneel in prayer and allow our sinful desires to die in repentance (Romans 12:1).

In the New Testament, the emphasis of God's covenant shifted from bodily circumcision to "circumcision of the heart." Baptism is the New Testament parallel to the Old Testament circumcision. Baptism cuts sin out of our lives. It is a spiritual circumcision that sets us apart as a child of God.

Baptism is our part of the spiritual covenant we enter into with God. Through baptism in Jesus' Name, we apply the blood of Jesus to our lives and hearts. Symbolically, it is a parallel to when the Israelites applied the blood of the sacrificial lamb to their doorposts to keep the death angel from visiting their home. Thank God for the blood of the Lamb, Christ Jesus, that covers my fractured, broken, and sinful humanity and gives me eternal life.

Colossians 2:11-12 KJV

In whom also ye are circumcised with the circumcision made without hands, in putting off the body of the sins of the flesh by the circumcision of Christ: Buried with him in baptism, wherein also ye are risen with him through the faith of the operation of God, who hath raised him from the dead.

Acts 22:16 KJV

And now why tarriest thou? Arise, and be baptized, and wash away thy sins, calling on the name of the Lord.

But It's Not That Spiritual

Today, we don't super-spiritualize a lot of the things we do in life. We go through our lives often living to please ourselves. I know that our choice toward cosmetic surgery has nothing to do with conscious rituals to "please the gods." We don't chant spiritual renditions over ourselves before we go into the operating room, though I'm sure many of us pray to the one true and living God, asking that the surgery go well and that we recover with no problems.

If the ancient people were to see our bodies lying on a surgical table of any kind, I'm sure their minds would go to an altar of sacrifice. In fact, there was a lot of superstition surrounding the "controversial" act of surgery in its beginnings. Doctors had to go underground to learn about the body. It was not acceptable to even cut open a dead body to learn about physical make-up. Doctors learned about the body in the darkness of night, a shrouded secret.[8]

I'm not painting the picture of the cosmetic surgery table as a place of blood and sacrifice to super-spiritualize it. I don't believe there are other-worldly spirits attached to everything we do. I do believe, however, that the choices we make are a part of our spiritual journey and show us the condition our hearts are in.

But there is a sacrifice of pain, time, recovery, and finances that goes into making a choice to have cosmetic surgery. There is a transitional time, and a growth period where we learn to accept ourselves and the changes made. There is after-care. We put a lot of ourselves into the choice to have surgery. It is a commitment

Does cosmetic surgery have anything to do with spirituality at all? I personally believe everything in life is connected to our spirituality. My leaning toward seeking spiritual perfectionism and religious performance is the same leaning that led me to cosmetic surgery. In both instances I wanted love and I thought I had to change myself in order to obtain that love. The truth is, God's love was there for me the whole time, unconditional, and without reserve.

The physical act of cosmetic surgery has spiritual implications—it comes down to the person and their inner experience of life. I am reminded of the popular quote, "It's not whether you win or lose, but how you play the game." In the same way, it's not whether you have surgery or not, but how you think about it that matters.

Even though I am not a sports-oriented person, let me use the only sports example I can think of. Tee-ball is connected to spirituality in that it teaches kids what it means to be a part of a team, to work together, and to support one another. It's not about the game itself. It's about showing up to the game, playing, having fun, and doing our best. When a parent attends their kids' sports games, it is about supporting the kid, building community, and being a part of something that is important in that kid's life.

Let's go back to the crooked teeth example. Does having crooked teeth impact a person spiritually? Does getting braces? The spiritual part is not about having crooked teeth or straight teeth. It is about having the confidence to be involved in life either way. If a person will never smile because they are ashamed of their crooked teeth, "shame" is the spiritual element they are living in. It isn't the crooked teeth, but the shame that is holding them back.

So what if a person really does have a physical flaw or abnormality? What if their teeth are crooked or their nose really is big? Should we expect them to be strong enough to be confidant no matter what, and never feel insecure? Of course not. We're only human. Still, I have to answer these questions with other questions. What's wrong with being imperfect? What's wrong with being real? What's wrong with accepting flaws and overlooking them? Why are we going to such lengths to rid ourselves of bodily flaws?

Maybe it's the same reason we go to such lengths to keep our life choices a secret from the church. We don't want to stand out, rock the boat, or receive judgment and rejection. Instead, we conform to cultural and religious expectations. We hide our physical flaws by covering them up, cutting them off, or adding onto them— just as we cover up our brokenness with religious performance, academic degrees, and high-profile occupations.

If you moved to a third world country next week, would you feel the need to change your body to fit in with the locals? Probably not. Would you have the capacity to experience the unconditional love and acceptance of the people around you, even though you were different? I think you would. It may take some effort and time, but eventually you would build relationships with the right people and positive things would happen.

There is no mold to make you worthy of giving and receiving love. You already are worthy. You don't have to be perfect, look perfect, or conform. You're worthy because God created you. Every one of us is worthy of love.

Cosmetic surgery may be the right choice for you. Like for me, it may catapult you into spiritual growth. But before you make that choice, please consider your life's blood and what you want to do with it.

Maybe cosmetic surgery isn't that serious to you. Maybe it's just like putting braces on your teeth. Either way, decide what your cosmetic choices mean to you, and consider the spiritual implications.

Questions for Reflection

- Do you think ancient practices have any bearing on current day happenings?
- Do you think body cutting is as serious today as it was throughout history? Why or why not?
- Is there any kind of spiritual brokenness involved in your choice concerning cosmetic surgery?
- Read Leviticus 19:27-28, Leviticus 21:5, and Jeremiah 7:29. These verses have to do with grieving. Do you think it is a natural human tendency to want to make an outward change after experiencing significant loss? Have you ever made a change to your body during grief?
- What kind of personal sacrifices are you willing to make to have cosmetic surgery?
- How will cosmetic surgery impact you spiritually?

Endnotes

1   Marx, Patricia. (2015). About Face: Why is South Korea the world's plastic surgery capital? *The New Yorker*. Accessed September 23, 2015 from www.newyorker.com/magazine/2015/03/23/about-face.

2   Shrayber, Mark. (2014). *Do-It-Yourself Plastic Surgery Leads to Devastating Results*. Jezebel.com

3   Kinnunen, T. (2010). 'A second youth': Pursuing happiness and respectability through cosmetic surgery in Finland. *Sociology Of Health & Illness*, 32(2), 258-271.

4   Strong's Concordance #1990

5   Jones, Bruce W. (no date). Cutting covenants and cutting animals: Biblical rituals and idioms. California State University. Accessed July 9, 2014. www.csub.edu/~bjones/cutdeal2.txt
6   Ibid.

7   Hunt, Michael (2006). The vow of the Nazirite. *Agape Bible Study*. Accessed July 9, 2014 on www.agapebiblestudy.com.

8   Dr. Richard Selzer. (1996). *Mortal Lessons: Notes on the Art of Surgery*. Harcourt Brace.

Finding Contentment

CHAPTER ELEVEN

Matthew 6:19-21 KJV

Lay not up for yourselves treasures upon earth, where moth and rust doth corrupt, and where thieves break through and steal: But lay up for yourselves treasures in heaven, where neither moth nor rust doth corrupt, and where thieves do not break through nor steal: For where your treasure is, there will your heart be also.

Unknowingly, I spent years in a discontented state. When the concept of contentment marched front and center into my mind and heart, my entire perspective on life changed. I stopped striving for control. I began to relax. Contentment is the state of being contented, satisfied, or having ease of mind.

When I started practicing contentment, I began to be satisfied with what I had. I say "practicing" because I haven't mastered the art of contentment. I still have days where I feel dreadfully discontent, but because I've been practicing contentment I am able to shift my mind into a state of gratefulness more easily. The journey to contentment is lifelong and ever-changing. Every time I round a bend, it seems like I am starting my quest for contentment all over again, but now it's easier to find my way back to that peaceful state of acceptance.

Contentment takes effort and time to develop. It doesn't come naturally, and it is not a fruit of the spirit. The fruit of the Spirit is love, joy, peace, long-suffering, gentleness, goodness, faith, meekness, and temperance (Galatians 5:22-23). At first, I wanted to lump contentment together with patience, but contentment and patience are not the same. We can patiently wait on what we want without being content. If we are still focused on what we want during our wait time, instead of being satisfied with what we have, we are not content. Maybe contentment is more a mix of patience, long-suffering, and peace.

At some point in our walk with God, if we keep growing, I believe we will all come to experience contentment. It is a place of gratefulness. No more longing. No more prayers full of begging God for something we want. No more desiring more or better for ourselves. Just simple thankfulness, rest, and contentment in God.

The King James Version of the Bible translates a few different Greek words into English words for "content" and "contentment." The Greek word *Arkeo* was translated into contentment in Luke 3:14, 1 Timothy 6:8, and Hebrews 13:5. The original definition of the word is very close to ours: "to be satisfied or contented with." But *Arkeo* takes the meaning of the word contentment to a new depth, described as: "to be sufficient, to possess sufficient strength, to be strong, to be enough for a thing."

Can you accept that you are "enough" to please the Lord? Can you picture yourself "possessing sufficient strength" to answer God's call, just as you are? Can you imagine being "strong enough" to be content with a body that you deem as less than perfect? With God's help, you can answer "yes" to each of these questions.

Discontentment
The First Step Toward Contentment

Discontentment is defined as "the state of dissatisfaction, lack of contentment, or malcontent." Synonyms include: uneasiness, inquietude, restlessness, and displeasure. In the Bible, the words *Mar* and *Marah,* translate to angry bitterness and discontent.

Recognizing you are discontent is not always a bad thing. In fact, God often uses discontentedness to move us from one place to another. If we were always satisfied, we would never grow, change, or step out in faith at all.

Remember the men in the Old Testament that joined David in the woods after he ran from King Saul? That story always makes me think of Robin Hood and the Merry Men. Four hundred men joined David, and the Bible describes them as "discontented" (1 Samuel 22:2).

Just as those discontented men stepped out and supported David, discontentment can push us to transform our world, to impact society for the good, and to change our culture. Good can come from discontentment, but only if we allow the negative frame of mind to move us forward into a positive one.

What happens when we are stuck in discontentment? That's the toxic place I was in before I made the choice to go forward with my surgery. It was a terrible season for me emotionally and spiritually.

I recently discovered a short book called *How To Be Totally Miserable*. The author, John Bytheway (by the way, what a cool last name for a writer), offered a 'self-hindering' list informing readers on the how-to's of staying miserable. Activities included: use your imagination to worry, relive your bad memories, blame everyone and everything, don't laugh or learn anything new, avoid prayer and Bible reading, and don't set goals. It's a sarcastically funny book, with a byproduct of teaching us how *not* to stay totally miserable.

Following suit, I've come up with five experiences I believe occur in the lives of people who are discontent. I call my list the "Five Cs of Discontentment" and they are: complaining, comparing, complacency, covetousness, and craving. If any of these "Five Cs" are in your life, you are likely discontent, and need to begin making changes to shift toward contentment.

The Five Cs of Discontentment

In discussing the Five Cs of Discontentment, I'll be focusing on ways we are discontent with our bodies, but you can apply these same ideas to any area of your life. We all experience discontentment, even if it comes in fleeting moments.

Often, discontentment is a result of unmet emotional or spiritual needs that end up manifesting through complaining, comparing, complacency, coveting, or craving. Recognizing we are discontent is the first step in figuring out what changes to make to care for our unmet needs.

Complaining

It's so easy to complain about our bodies. We can complain that our bodies are ugly, or fat, or flat, or the wrong color, or the wrong shape. When we complain about our bodies we are essentially speaking curses over ourselves. We can drive ourselves insane with the negativity that accompanies complaining.

We don't have to keep complaining. We can make a choice to stop complaining, but that is just the first step. It's not enough to stop verbalizing our complaints if we don't do something to work on the thought patterns behind the complaints.

Look deeper inside. Is there anything else in your life you are unhappy with besides your body? Are complaints the result of you transferring emotions from another issue onto your body? Transferring emotions onto your body is similar to implosive anger, where you're angry at another person or situation but take it out on yourself. Are you genuinely complaining about your body, or are you using your body as a distraction from other issues you'd rather not face?

Comparing

If we are discontent, we will compare ourselves to the people around us, or to the person we used to be. We will believe what we have isn't as good as what someone else has, or what we had in the past. We will verbalize the differences between our bodies and other people's bodies. We will often complain along with comparing.

Our comparisons are often not based on reality. When we compare ourselves to others, we don't know the truth about another person's situation or circumstance. The Bible warns us against comparing ourselves to others: "... *They measuring themselves by themselves, and comparing themselves among themselves, are not wise*" (2 Corinthians 10:12 KJV).

Instead of comparing our bodies, we can learn from and support each other. If you want your body to be healthy or more fit, start hanging out with people that exercise. Learn from them. Transform your body from the inside out, starting with your thoughts and what you eat. It's not wrong to look to another person or our previous condition for inspiration, but we don't want to stay stuck in comparison.

Complacency

Complacency is a dangerous place to come to in our discontent. It may be even more dangerous than complaining, comparing, coveting, or craving. Complacency disguises itself as contentment, but in reality we are so discontent that we give up seeking growth and change, and we begin to find our satisfaction in the temporary things of this life.

Complacency is "a feeling of quiet pleasure or security, often while unaware of some potential danger, defect, or the like; self-satisfaction or smug satisfaction with an existing situation, or condition." Complacency is dangerous because it gives a false sense of contentment and satisfaction, instead of true contentment, which we find in God.

When we are lost in complacency, our discontent doesn't push us to be mighty women of valor, as it did with the men who joined David's army. Instead, we settle for whatever satisfies the flesh at the moment. I found myself in complacency in the months after my cosmetic surgery.

It was a time when I was distracted with the newness of my body change. It was also a time when a lot of other exciting things were happening in my life. I thought I was content because I wasn't complaining, comparing, coveting, or craving. But I also wasn't resting in God. I was filling my life with other distractions—like relationships, religious performance, and education.

Complacency was a part of my journey to contentment. Thankfully, I continued to move forward out of complacency, but when I started experiencing the Five Cs again, I knew the discontentment hadn't left. I had just covered it up for a while.

Covetousness

Discontentment comes down to one sin—a sin that was so rampant, God issued the 10th Commandment against it: coveting (lust). The 10th Commandment is found in Exodus 20:17 KJV, "*You shall not covet your neighbor's house; you shall not covet your neighbor's wife, or his male servant, or his female servant, or his ox, or his donkey, or anything that is your neighbor's.*"

Jude 1:16 ESV says, "*These are grumblers, malcontents, following their own sinful desires; they are loud-mouthed boasters, showing favoritism to gain advantage.*" The same verse in the NLT puts it this way, "*These people are grumblers and complainers, living only to satisfy their desires. They brag loudly about themselves, and they flatter others to get what they want.*"

Covetous people want what other people have. When we experience covetousness, we think our lives would be better if we had what "they" have. It's different than comparing because you secretly want another person's situation or circumstance to be your own, even if you don't complain about your own situation, or outline the differences through logically comparing.

Sometimes, covetousness shows itself in the form of vicarious living. When you live vicariously through another person, you experience thoughts and feelings as if their actions were your own. It can happen as you watch a movie, scroll through Facebook, or as you listen to your friend's stories about their lives. If you are experiencing life through someone else, you may be living in a state of covetousness even if you are not consciously thinking that you want what they have in life.

Hebrews 13:5 KJV

Let your conversation be without covetousness; and be content with such things as ye have: for he hath said, I will never leave thee, nor forsake thee.

Craving

What happens in the physical body when we have a craving? We become antsy, or restless. A craving starts like an itch that begins to consume our thoughts, and we can't stop thinking about the object of our desire. Eventually, the restlessness will return, even after we get what we are longing for. The craving experience is common with addicts and alcoholics, but also occurs when a person is discontent.

The "itch" happens when we crave something that we are addicted to. It happens in our spirit and mind when we lust after the things that we want—be it a relationship, beauty, ideal identity, youthfulness, love, success, money, or anything really. If you allow your cravings to lead your life, you may end up making choices based on a want or longing, instead of making a well thought out decision. People who live to fulfill their cravings walk after their own lusts. They are sensual, or concerned with pleasing the five senses: taste, touch, smell, sight, and sound.

2 Timothy 4:3-4 NLT says, *"For a time is coming when people will no longer listen to sound and wholesome teaching. They will follow their own desires and will look for teachers who will tell them whatever their itching ears want to hear. They will reject the truth and chase after myths."*

The myth you chase is a lie that tells you that what you crave will satisfy your itch. Chasing the myth means you're rejecting truth. Who are you listening to? Whose teaching have you blocked from your ears? Are you living to satisfy a craving?

When you experience the "itching" feeling—the anxiety, lust, desire, craving, and discontent—turn to God. Seek Him for contentment. Rest in His peace and let God fulfill your heart's desperate desires. If we hunger for the things of the Spirit, God will meet our true needs, and we will drink from the water that will finally quench our craving thirst (John 4:14). Seek the Lord, resist the devil, pursue righteousness and peace, and God will strengthen your heart (Isaiah 55:6, James 4:7, Psalm 34:14, Psalm 27:14).

Contentment – You Are Enough!

I think it is safe to say we all want to move out of discontentment into contentment. We have two options. We can either: 1. Stay discontented, or 2. Change our thought patterns and make a shift in the way we think and live. We can move out of a state of discontentment, but we have to make a conscious choice to practice contentment, and ask the Lord for His help.

The transition to contentment is separate from a choice about cosmetic surgery. Choosing to go forward with cosmetic surgery won't automatically remove discontent from your life. Choosing not to go forward also won't remove the discontent. Your cosmetic considerations can impede or progress your developmental process, but it all depends on your perspective.

Your journey to contentment will have ups and downs. You will face challenges and eventually overcome them. There will be pain. There will be healing. There will be disappointments and victories.

The journey to contentment is full of choices and consequences. Unexpected plot twists will happen. You may choose surgery, and you may not; life will move forward either way and you will still have to do the hard work to grow.

Self-Esteem

A while ago, I was thinking about the way many churches approach teaching young people about self-esteem. I've heard many people say that we shouldn't have "self-esteem," but we should have "God-esteem." I know what these people are trying to communicate—God is our source and our lives revolve around Him, not ourselves. I think the people who say such things are well-meaning and trying to teach principles of humility. But as the wise C.S. Lewis once wrote, "True humility is not thinking less of yourself, but thinking of yourself less."

I believe we should have healthy self-esteem—not self worship—self-esteem. The definition of self-esteem is "confidence in one's own worth or abilities; self-respect." Sadly, I've met a number of Christians who equate self-esteem, or self-respect, with the sin of pride. Respecting yourself is not prideful, it's being a good steward of the life, body, and emotions God gave you.

It's not prideful to care for your mental, emotional, and spiritual health. It's good stewardship. Your body is the temple of the Holy Ghost. It's your responsibility to take care of the everything God has given you.

God created you and loves you. He made you with a purpose, and you need to respect yourself. To disrespect yourself is to disrespect your Creator. Would you stand back and do nothing if a vandal entered your church and started destroying it? No. Would you allow someone to interrupt a church service with criticism from the audience? No. So why would you allow harm to your body, or allow negative thoughts to consume your mind?

I've heard Christian youth leaders teach young people that they should accept themselves as they are "because God created them." That there "shouldn't" be an element of complaint or comparison, and that they "should" accept their body as is "because God made them that way." That line of thinking reminds me of a parent that tells a child what to do "because I said so" without teaching about principles.

I don't think God expects us to fully appreciate every aspect of our bodies all of the time. It is okay to admit the truth if we don't like something about ourselves. That's called honesty, and God is all about honesty. We aren't going to hurt God's feelings by admitting there is something about our bodies we don't like too much.

Even if you do pursue cosmetic surgery, there will be a part of your body that you don't fully appreciate at some point down the road. Just because we don't like a situation, doesn't mean we can't eventually come to a place of acceptance and contentment—with or without cosmetic surgery. Contentment is the ultimate goal, no matter what choice you make in this season of your life.

But I'm Not _____ Enough

Too many of us are living in a place of inadequacy. We fall into a trap of thinking we can't find contentment, make a positive difference in the world, or fully live because we aren't _____ enough. You fill in the blank. Maybe you are like I was, thinking you aren't good enough, pretty enough, or cool and fun enough.

But you are. You are enough.

At some point in our lives, most everyone will feel inadequate. We are not alone in our feelings of not being "enough." Many people in the Bible experienced feelings of inadequacy, and God never once condemned them for feeling that way. Instead, He confirmed each person, and made sure they knew they were in His presence, and accepted as they were.

When God called Moses to lead the children of Israel out of slavery, Moses asked the question, "Who am I that I should go?" (Exodus 3:11) When God called Gideon to save His people from the Midianites, Gideon's response was, "Oh, Lord, how can I? My family is the least, and I am the youngest" (Judges 6:15). When God called Jeremiah to be a prophet, his response was, "I cannot speak: for I am a child" (Jeremiah 1:6).

There's a unique theme that emerges in the scriptures every time a person voiced their feelings of inadequacy to God. His response was the same: He would go with them, He would give them the words they were to say, and He would not leave them. They were not to focus on their own inadequacy, but instead to find their confidence in God's presence. Note: God didn't say they weren't inadequate. He wanted them to go forward despite inadequacy. He wanted them to go forward so He could be their strength.

When Moses expressed self-doubt, God told Moses He would *certainly be with him*. Moses went to Egypt to lead the people out of bondage not because He was a strong leader, but because God was with him and leading him (Exodus 3:12-14).

When Gideon expressed his feelings of inadequacy, God told Gideon He was with him and that the Army would have victory. Judges 6:16 says, *"And the Lord said unto him,* **Surely I will be with thee,** *and thou shalt smite the Midianites as one man."*

When Jeremiah said he wasn't "old enough" to speak, God came against Jeremiah's thought process. He put His own words into the young man's mouth. Look at what Jeremiah 1:4-9 NLT says.

> *The Lord gave me this message: "I knew you before I formed you in your mother's womb. Before you were born I set you apart and appointed you as my prophet to the nations."*
> *"O Sovereign Lord," I said, "I can't speak for you! I'm too young!"*
> *The Lord replied, "Don't say, 'I'm too young,' for you must go wherever I send you and say whatever I tell you. And don't be afraid of the people, for I will be with you and protect you. I, the Lord, have spoken! Then the Lord reached out and touched my mouth and said, "Look, I have put my words in your mouth!"*

God Has a Plan

Just like He had a plan for Jeremiah, God has a plan for our lives. He has a plan to use us despite our limitations. When I'm feeling unsure or inadequate, I pray this prayer: "Lord, please give me the peace and strength to do Your will." That 'peace and strength' can only come from one source, and it isn't from our looks, our personality, or our knowledge. It comes from God alone.

Earlier, we learned about the Greek word *Arkeo*, "to be satisfied or contented with, to be sufficient, to possess sufficient strength, to be strong, to be enough for a thing . . ." There is another Greek word, *Autarkes*, which means "competence, sufficiency and satisfaction, needing no assistance, or content." *Autarkes* translates to "sufficiency" in 2 Corinthians 9:8.

2 Corinthians 9:8

*And God is able to make all grace abound toward you, that you, always having all **sufficiency** in all things, may have an abundance for every good work.*

Grace abounds in our imperfections. Jesus makes up for our lack. We show His strength through our weaknesses. In Christ Jesus, you have what it takes to accomplish God's plan for your life. You are sufficient—enough—to follow Him, regardless of how inadequate you may feel.

Our Christian walk is not about us. It's not about the way we look, or how smart we are, or what others think of us. It's all about Jesus and sharing the Gospel with the world. When you are filled with the Holy Spirit of God, you are enough—contented, sufficient—to make a positive difference in the world. God says you are content—enough, sufficient—in your frailty and imperfection. In Christ Jesus, you are content—enough!

2 Corinthians 3:5
Not that we are sufficient of ourselves to think any thing as of ourselves; but our sufficiency is of God.

Questions for Reflection

- Do you practice contentment or discontentment?
- Do you engage in one of the Five Cs of Discontentment?
- Discontentment can move you toward contentment by motivating you to make changes in your life. In what ways can you see your life changing for the better because of acknowledging discontent?
- Do you believe God is ready to step into your life, despite any feelings of inadequacy, and empower you to do His work?
- Read Philippians 4:13 and Joshua 1:9. After learning about contentment and sufficiency, do these verses take on new meaning for you?
- Finding contentment isn't about having perfect self-esteem, or liking every part of your life or your body. It is about knowing that you are enough in Christ. Every day, speak the following affirmation over yourself: In Jesus I am sufficient. I am enough. I am content.

Beautifully Created

CHAPTER TWELVE

Ecclesiastics 3:11 ESV
He has made everything beautiful in its time.

God's love isn't like human love. Human love is limited and often dependent on various criteria to be met before it is given or received. God doesn't love like we love.

God doesn't love us more when we are physically healthy than He does when we are sick. He doesn't love us less if we are emotionally wounded and struggling to function than He does when we are at our best and happiest.

God doesn't increase His love for us when we accomplish great things, and He doesn't withdrawal His love from us when we make mistakes. God knows our frailty. He has compassion toward us.

I can testify to the unfailing love of God. He's faithful when I'm not. He's forgiving when I'm bitter. He sees my worth and dwells in me. He fills me with His Spirit over and over again. In the midst of my darkest times of brokenness and pain, He has never left me. He's continually re-creating me, renewing me, and giving me strength.

He accepted me when I was a desperate young girl with a hole in my heart. He filled me with His love. He still completes me.

With Jesus, I am enough. I am content. I have what it takes to accomplish His will.

I am not perfect. I've made choices that conflict with my own convictions. I have many flaws. But I am here, and I offer myself to the Lord for use in His kingdom. I love Him and He loves me.

God created me. God created you. He created the beautiful, imperfect me and you. He created the world we were born into. He set up the system that brought us into being. He designed our fingerprints and marked us individually.

Psalms 139:13-14

You created me. You knitted me together like a woman knits a scarf. I praise You because You took the time to make me. From the depths of my soul, now I know how amazing Your creations is.

As the creative person God made me to be, I enjoy all types of art. I paint, sew, draw pictures, and make pottery. I'm not the best artist or craftiest person, but I enjoy expressing myself through art. I usually give my art away as gifts to friends and family.

A few years ago, I decided to learn to knit. I bought thick yarn in various colors, two fat knitting needles, and the *Knitting for Dummies* book. For the next two years, my friends and family received scarves for Christmas. I made long scarves with yarn fringe and matching pin-on flowers. They were warm, fun, and unique for each person.

My scarves weren't perfect. I made them out of love and I did my best, but if a professional knitter were to look over my work,

I have no doubt they would easily find flaws. The thing is, I never learned to pearl, only to knit. Personally, I think the scarves turned out cute, despite the fact that all the knits were on one side and all the pearls on the other.

I remember praying as I knitted. I prayed for the people that would wear my scarf-gifts. I gained satisfaction when I saw them open their presents and see their scarf, made in their favorite color. Not one person that received a scarf looked it over and pointed out the uneven knots I tied. None of them examined the handmade flowers and told me how the petals were uneven, or how my stitches didn't match. In fact, it was the imperfection of the item that made my creation beautiful.

When God makes a flower, the petals He creates aren't aesthetically "perfect" either. Each flower petal is different than the next. Each part is vulnerable, easily torn.

God makes people the way He makes flowers. When God makes people, He makes us imperfect. Most of us have one leg that's slightly longer than the other. Each side of the body is usually not a perfect reflection of the other side.

Sometimes, a gene mutation causes our imperfections. Sometimes our imperfections come when our vulnerability meets trauma. We become scarred by a car accident. We loose mobility after we break a bone. One side of our face droops due to pressure on the nerves in our brain after a stroke. We are imperfect, vulnerable, beautifully created flowers.

Can you imagine an animal complaining about the color of its fur? Animals don't have the ability to be critical or complain about imperfections. What if a corn-cob complained that its rows of kernels were not evenly spaced? It would be ridiculous. God's creation brings Him glory just by being what it is. Our family dogs bring glory to God as the Creator simply by running across the yard barking at squirrels. They are being themselves—dogs—living life, having fun, and being what God created them to be!

Romans 9:20-21 NLT

Should the thing that was created say to the one who created it, "Why have you made me like this?"[1] When a potter makes jars out of clay, doesn't he have a right to use the same lump of clay to make one jar for decoration and another to throw garbage into?

Isaiah 45:9-10 NLT

What sorrow awaits those who argue with their Creator.
Does a clay pot argue with its maker?
Does the clay dispute with the one who shapes it, saying,
'Stop, you're doing it wrong!' Does the pot exclaim,
'How clumsy can you be?' How terrible it would be if a
newborn baby said to its father, 'Why was I born?'
or if it said to its mother, 'Why did you make me this way?'

Can you imagine if your art project complained to you about how you made it? That's essentially what we do to God when we complain about our bodies and how He made us. But we're human, imperfect, and we complain.

The problem isn't about ever having a complaint. The problem is that some of us don't appreciate anything about the way God made us. We only see the flaws. We focus on what we don't like about our bodies instead of focusing on God. Yet God loves us, despite our complaints.

Psalm 119:73 KJV

Your hands have made me and fashioned me;
Give me understanding, that I may learn Your commandments.

Learning God's commandments takes time. I don't mean learning to recite them, but learning to live them out. It takes time to learn not to covet. When it comes to our bodies, the Tenth Commandment could be translated to: "Don't wish your body was like their bodies. Don't wish your nose had been shaped like their noses. Don't wish your shape were larger or smaller." In our humanity, some of us will have a real struggle to find contentment and stop longing for something we don't have.

I've experienced the struggle. I have shared my struggle with you. I know what it is to be out of control with negative thinking, wishing my body were more beautiful. I was bound to the sin of covetousness, which kept me from living life with contented confidence. I was consumed by the feeling that I wasn't good enough. For many years I felt unworthy, because I was believing a lie and chasing a beauty myth.

The Greek word for sin is *"hamartia."* It's an archery term meaning "to miss the mark," or to miss hitting the bull's-eye. I love how Paul used archery as an example in Philippians 3:14. He encourages us to "keep pressing toward the mark of the high calling of Christ Jesus." That mark—that high calling—it's the bull's-eye of a target called the Christian life.

I've always been at peace with the fact that I'm not into sports. I've never felt the need to compete or perform athletically. I have never found my worth in whether or not I can hit a bull's-eye using a bow and arrow, but I enjoy trying. I've learned not to expect perfection out of myself, and that God doesn't expect perfection out of me either.

We are sinners. That's why Jesus died. If we had the ability to be perfect, He would have never had to come to save us. The Bible says that Jesus understands all of our temptations, feelings, and struggles (Hebrews 4:15). Jesus knows what it is like to feel ugly. He knows what it is like to be rejected because of the way He looked.

In Isaiah 53:2-3 KJV, the prophecy is clear: "*. . . He hath no form nor comeliness; and when we shall see him, there is no beauty that we should desire him. He is despised and rejected of men; a man of sorrows, and acquainted with grief: and we hid as it were our faces from him; he was despised, and we esteemed him not.*"

I think a lot about Jesus. I wouldn't be surprised if He had a big nose. I am confidant that He wasn't obsessed with His looks. He unselfishly didn't care about His looks as He fulfilled his purpose, carrying every bit of my sin and shame to the cross. He died, naked and vulnerable, beaten bloody, deformed and disfigured through abusive trauma imposed on Him. Yet He went to the cross for me, and for you.

Isaiah 53:4-5 KJV continues, *"Surely he hath borne our griefs, and carried our sorrows: yet we did esteem him stricken, smitten of God, and afflicted. But he was wounded for our transgressions, he was bruised for our iniquities: the chastisement of our peace was upon him; and with his stripes we are healed."*

We hid our faces from the trauma. It reminded us of our vulnerability. It could have been us on the cross.

Jesus suffered and died for us. He suffered and died for me. There was a time in my life where I didn't believe that Jesus would have come and died just for me alone. I believed He came for all of humanity, but for *me*? It was difficult to accept that kind of love on a personal level. I knew that God so loved the world, but I didn't know that God so loved *me*.

It was a Sunday church service, and I remember standing at the front of the sanctuary with a lot of other people as we prayed after the message. The pastor finished preaching a sermon about the unconditional love of God. I looked across the church and saw a young woman about my age. She was obviously touched by the presence of God. I could sense how much God loved her.

And then I had an epiphany that as much as God loved her, He loved me too. The idea that God loved me as much as He loved the people around me was overwhelming. The realization of God's love for me was an incredible experience.

The love He has for me He has for us all. What He has done for me, He will do for you. He loves you just as you are, with every choice you make. Yes, even when you sin.

We fall short and miss the mark in many areas of life, and every time God is there to pick us up and carry us the rest of the way. No matter what sin we struggle with—whether it's vanity, feelings of low self-worth, pride, comparing ourselves to others, taking matters into our own hands, and many other sins—His grace is sufficient to help us grow through our issues and draw us closer to Him. I'm so thankful for His grace and love, and that He's not leaving me to die in my sin.

As we walk in grace toward maturity in our faith, it's important to look into our hearts with honesty and identify what motivates us to make choices about the way we live our lives. Why are you considering cosmetic surgery? What is the state of your heart? What direction is the target of God's high calling on your life? What direction is your arrow aiming?

When I first started thinking about cosmetic surgery, I felt a burst of confidence as if I had found the answer to my problems. I was distracted for several months by the idea of my coming transformation. For weeks after the surgery, I was preoccupied with recovery. I slept a lot, took pain medication, tended to my stitches, and waited for the swelling to go down in my nose and chin. At first, it was impossible to tell what the end result would look like.

As the swelling went down, it took time for me to accept the changes I saw in the mirror. As my new face began to emerge, my altered nose wasn't perfect. My old feelings began waking back up. I realized that in my heart nothing had changed. The distraction of the "new me" had to end, so I could begin to work on the real issues I had ignored and start the inner growth I desperately needed.

It took undergoing cosmetic surgery to wake me up to the truth I had to face in myself. It was during those months of adjustment that I unconditionally accepted myself for the first time. I was seventeen when I learned that changing the outside didn't change my inside experience of life.

With quiet desperation, I sought God with many tears. I poured my soul out to Him and He poured His Spirit into me. The first two years after my surgery I spent hours in prayer, alone with God. I felt deep emotional closeness to God. By the leading of God's Spirit and through the power of His Word, I began to work through my feelings of unworthiness and come to accept myself as His beautiful creation. I am humbled at how God brought victory into my soul.

As I practice accepting my imperfections without criticism, my "grace muscles" become stronger. The more love and grace I have for myself, the more I am able to show love and grace to others. The capacity to unconditionally love is the greatest beauty there is.

As you go forward into the next season of your life, with whatever choices you make, with whatever consequences may come, I pray you would go with love and grace. Give yourself grace to make mistakes and to learn from them. Love yourself, God's creation, with all of your flaws and imperfections.

Read the Word of God. Pray. Seek the Lord. Allow Him to lead you. He is gentle and kind. You are made in His image. Be gentle and kind to yourself.

Romans 14:22 NLT

You may believe there's nothing wrong with what you are doing, but keep it between yourself and God. Blessed are those who don't feel guilty for doing something they have decided is right.

Happy is the man who does not condemn himself in the thing which he allows.

Questions for Reflection

- Do you feel the love of God in your life?
- Think about God's creation in nature. Do you notice the imperfections, or the beauty?
- When you think of God as your Creator, how does that make you feel? Do you have any bitterness or resentment toward God and the way He made you?
- In what ways do you "miss the mark" and sin? Do you feel God loves you less because you can't hit the center of the bull's-eye?
- What is your personal response toward yourself when you sin? Do you treat yourself with love and respect, which leads to repentance? Or do you treat yourself with condemnation and self-hatred, which leads to low self-esteem?

- Have you ever considered what Jesus looked like? How does it make you feel when you think about Jesus understanding feelings of inadequacy and rejection?
- Do you believe Jesus died to save *you*?
- Study Romans Chapter 14. How does this chapter relate to the current cultural inclinations about cosmetic surgery?
- Focus on Romans 14:22. You will allow many things in your life, some things people will understand, and other things people won't understand. What matters is your faith in God, and how you stand before Him. Do you feel content in Christ concerning your decision about cosmetic surgery? If not, do you believe you can shift from a state of condemnation to blessed happiness?
- Just as you practice contentment, practice grace and love. Internalize God's grace and love toward yourself, so that you can in turn give grace and love to the people in your life.
- Say this affirmation: *I am not perfect, but Jesus loves me. He died in my place. He gives me grace to keep pressing toward the mark. I will love others and give them grace to be imperfect. I will love myself unconditionally, as God loves me, so that I can love others as I love myself.*

Afterword

As a millennial, I feel compelled to write about issues unique to the current generation. I want to seek out the Christian response to the concerns we face. Today's world can be difficult to navigate, even with God and His Word guiding us one step at a time.

I believe the majority of the older generation does not have a full understanding of the psychological struggles younger generations face. I've talked to some older ministers who are at a loss for how to face current controversies. They often answer our questions with religious tradition, and not with experience or wisdom because they grew up in a simpler time.

Our generation is complicated. It doesn't help if we as Christians stick our heads in the sand, afraid to learn, afraid to listen, and afraid to seek out an effective response. Those of us in the midst of making decisions pertaining to this generation have a choice to follow our hearts and pursue what we want because we can, or to seek out Biblical principles to apply to the situation.

I believe we are to seek the Lord and to educate ourselves. Let's dig deep inside, into prayer, into the Bible, and into research. What are other people saying? What is our heart saying? What Biblical principles apply? What is God saying?

Dialogue starts with empathy. I believe we can be secure enough to have hard conversations, and to listen without judgment, or self-defense. If we listen to each other, then we have a better chance at reaching victory in Jesus together.

Thank you for reading my story and what I've learned. I don't have all the answers, and I don't know your situation, but I hope my book was a place for you to start sorting through questions. I pray you will invite Jesus into your heart and into your decision-making process.

♡ Rachael

About the Author

Rachael Kathleen Hartman loves Jesus, reading, and writing. She enjoys learning about different cultures, meeting new people, and traveling with her two dapple dachshunds, Danny and Darla.

She has an MS in Human Services with a Specialization in Counseling, a BA in Liberal Studies with a Minor in Writing, and is a certified Life Coach. Prior to secular college, she spent two and a half years in Bible College as a Theology Major.

Rachael grew up as a proud ARMY BRAT. She was born in Houston, Texas and then moved a lot: Fort Hood, Texas; Goppingen, Germany; Fort Dix, New Jersey; Fort Sheridan, Illinois; back to Fort Hood, Texas; Annandale, Virginia; Silver Spring, Maryland; Fort Stewart, Georgia; and Fort Bragg, North Carolina. As a young adult, she's lived in Texas, Louisiana, and Georgia.

She is the author of three books, including *Angel: The True Story of an Undeserved Chance* (2013), *Called to Write, Chosen to Publish: Inspiration for Christian Writers* (2015), and *Facing Myself: An Introspective Look at Cosmetic Surgery* (2016).

In 2013, she started Our Written Lives of Hope and offering publishing services to independent authors. Rachael specializes in coaching aspiring authors. She also speaks to groups about writing and living for Jesus.

RachaelKathleenHartman.com
OurWrittenLives.com

other books by Rachael Kathleen Hartman

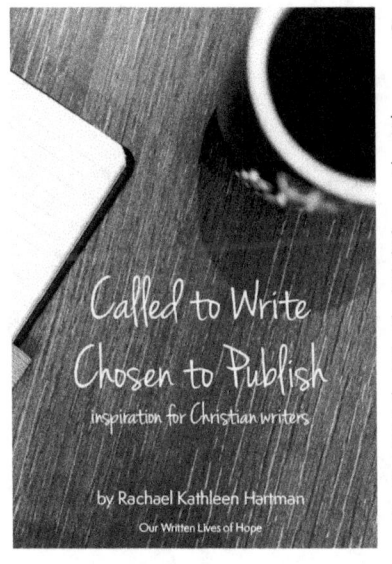

Called to Write, Chosen to Publish

20 inspirational and scripture-based thoughts for Christian writers.

"Write, even if millions of people have access to the words, but only hundreds read it. Write, even if writing bares your soul, and you're left alone and exposed. Write, for your life was meant to bring the hope of Christ to those who know and read it. And so, God provides Our Written Lives of Hope..."

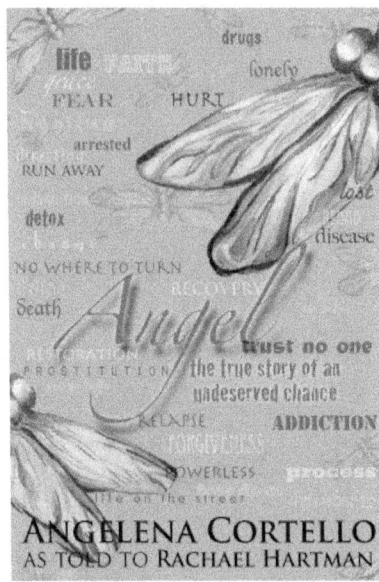

Angel: The True Story of an Undeserved Chance

Rachael writes and shares Angel Cortello's testimony story. Angel was once on the streets, addicted to drugs, and lost in a world of emotional problems. This is the true story of how God delivered Angel, and the lessons she learned during recovery. Topics include: drugs, street life, prostitution, jail, addiction recovery, HIV, Bi-Polar Disorder, integration back into church, and life lessons after deliverance.

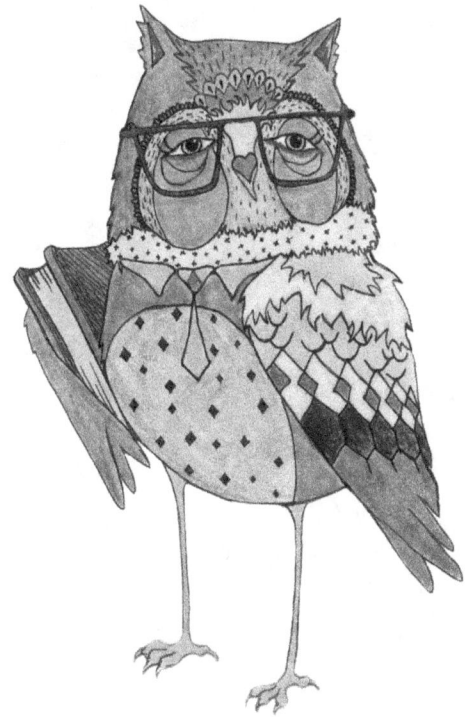

Our Written Lives
book publishing services
www.owlofhope.com

www.ingramcontent.com/pod-product-compliance
Lightning Source LLC
Chambersburg PA
CBHW052022290426
44112CB00014B/2339